Drugs for children

World Health Organization
Regional Office for Europe
Copenhagen

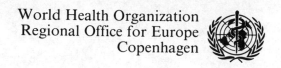

Drugs for children

ICP/DSE 102/s05

Drugs for children / [editor-in-chief: G. Rylance]
Copenhagen : WHO. Regional Office for Europe, 1987
185p. ISBN 92-890-1048-7
Drug Utilization — Child

ISBN 92 890 1048 7

Editor-in-Chief

Dr G. Rylance

Consultant in Paediatric Clinical Pharmacology, The Children's Hospital, Birmingham, United Kingdom

Principal Contributors

Dr N.D. Barnes

Department of Paediatrics, Addenbrooke's Hospital, Cambridge, United Kingdom

Dr A.W. Craft

Department of Child Health, Royal Victoria Infirmary, Newcastle-upon-Tyne, United Kingdom

Dr R. George

The Children's Hospital, Birmingham, United Kingdom

Professor A.D. Milner

Department of Child Health, University of Nottingham, United Kingdom

Acknowledgements

The following people are gratefully acknowledged for their help and advice in the preparation of the text:

Professor M. Albani
Universitäts-Kinderklinik
Hamburg
Federal Republic of Germany

Dr C. Bakoula
Institute of Child Health
Aghia Sophia Children's Hospital
Athens
Greece

Professor F. Bläker
Deutsche Gesellschaft für
  Kinderheilkunde
Hamburg
Federal Republic of Germany

Professor L. Boréus
Department of Clinical
  Pharmacology
Karolinska Hospital
Stockholm
Sweden

Professor E. Gladtke
Universitäts-Kinderklinik
Cologne
Federal Republic of Germany

Professor M. Hassar
Professeur de pharmacologie
  clinique
Faculté de médecine
Rabat
Morocco

Professor G. Heimann
Head, Department of Paediatrics
Technical University
Aachen
Federal Republic of Germany

Dr H.M. Lenicker
Karin Grech Hospital
Malta

Professor G. Lenoir
Service de pédiatrie générale
Département de pédiatrie
Hôpital Necker Enfants
  Malades
Paris
France

Professor D. Mardesic
Hospital Centre for Sick
  Children
Zagreb
Yugoslavia

Professor D. Reinhardt
Universitäts-Kinderklinik
Düsseldorf
Federal Republic of Germany

Dr P. Sampedro
Children's Hospital for the
  Social Security System
Barcelona
Spain

Professor H.J. Seyberth
Universitäts-Kinderklinik
Heidelberg
Federal Republic of Germany

Professor V. Spicak
Head, Paediatric Department
Bulovka Hospital
Prague
Czechoslovakia

Valuable assistance was also received from:

Dr M. Bonati
Milan
Italy

Dr K. Méhes
Györ
Hungary

Dr E.A. Cachia
Ta' Xbiex
Malta

Dr A. Mifsud
G'Mangia
Malta

Dr T. Chambers
Bristol
United Kingdom

Dr Brigita Radeva
Sofia
Bulgaria

Dr P. Cholnoky
Szombathely
Hungary

Dr D. Schuler
Budapest
Hungary

Dr E. Cserháti
Budapest
Hungary

Professor S. Doxiadis
Athens
Greece

Dr L. Greco
Naples
Italy

Dr I. Szórády
Szeged
Hungary

Dr K. Jährig
Greifswald
German Democratic Republic

Dr Anne Träger
Jena
German Democratic Republic

Professor K. Kerrebijn
Rotterdam
Netherlands

Dr S. Yaffe
Bethesda
United States of America

Editorial coordinator

Ms Inga Lunde
Pharmaceuticals
WHO Regional Office for Europe
Copenhagen
Denmark

CONTENTS

Introduction

This guide aims to outline the principles and problems of drug use in children and to help physicians increase their appreciation and knowledge of specific problem areas. The aspects of drug use that relate specifically to hospital practice, and some that raise no problems in paediatric practice, have been omitted. This is, therefore, not a textbook of paediatric pharmacology or therapeutics, but a handbook on safe and effective therapy primarily for the physician prescribing for children outside hospitals. It is not intended to include problems relating to specialist newborn practice.

Children differ from adults in the way that they handle and respond to drugs. There is also great variation among children of different ages. These differences may persist even when dosage is adjusted for body weight or surface area.

Safe and effective therapy in children should in theory result if prescribing is based on data obtained for a particular age group and disease. Although development proceeds in a predictable fashion in any given child, individuals still vary widely. The physician must therefore anticipate variation in drug handling and response.

These differences between and within individuals render the rational use of drugs more difficult in children than in adults.

An attempt has been made to describe current orthodox therapeutic practice. Variations in national practice have necessitated some modification and compromise. Some drugs are not available in all countries and other equally effective drugs that are similar to those mentioned in this text may well be more commonly used in some countries. Nevertheless, it is not possible to satisfy everyone and the text is based on drugs available in most countries.

The book is divided into two parts, the first dealing with prescribing principles and therapeutic approaches and the second with specific drug groups and clinical problems.

Drug doses are stated in their most practical form. In most cases a dose is specified for three age bands: less than 1 year, 1–4 years and 5–12 years. Children over 12 years old generally receive an adult dose. Decimal points for numerals less than unity have usually been omitted by expressing doses as whole numbers of a smaller mass unit; thus

1

0.01 ml is described as $10\,\mu l$ and 0.5–1 mg is described as $500\,\mu g$–1 mg. Where doses are more appropriately expressed in relation to body weight or surface area, the total daily dose and number of divided doses is indicated. Centile charts for weight are shown in Fig. 1 and 2. Dose frequency is stated as number of doses per day, unless there are specific reasons to specify the interval between doses in hours.

The drug names used in this book are the international nonproprietary names (INN) for pharmaceutical substances proposed or recommended by WHO,[a] which may differ slightly from those that appear in the British Pharmacopoeia. Where they differ markedly, the British Pharmacopoeia name has been added in parentheses.

Similarly, the names of diseases are those recommended by the Council for International Organizations of Medical Sciences (CIOMS) and WHO in the International Nomenclature of Diseases.[b]

[a] *International nonproprietary names (INN) for pharmaceutical substances.* Cumulative list No. 6. Geneva, World Health Organization, 1982.

[b] *International nomenclature of diseases. Vol. II. Infectious diseases.* Geneva, CIOMS, 1982 (Part 2), 1983 (Part 3), 1985 (Part 1).

Fig. 1. Centile chart of weight for girls, showing 10th, 50th and 90th centiles

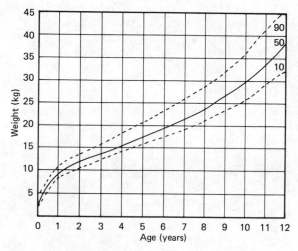

Source: Adapted from **Tanner, J.M. & Whitehouse, R.H.** *Growth and development record.* Twickenham, Printwell Press Ltd., 1959.

Fig. 2. Centile chart of weight for boys, showing 10th, 50th and 90th centiles

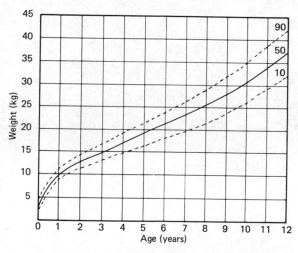

Source: Adapted from **Tanner, J.M. & Whitehouse, R.H.** *Growth and development record.* Twickenham, Printwell Press Ltd., 1959.

3

Problems with drug therapy in children

Prescribing for children presents many problems that often interact. These are examined in more detail later but may be outlined under three headings:

— child and family
— drugs
— the prescriber.

Child and family

The state of the child's growth and development affects drug handling and response. Doses may be unpredictable owing to variability in drug kinetics and dynamics.

Compliance with therapy involves at least two people, parent and child, and often more. This complicates the process and increases the chances of error.

Parents usually have inadequate knowledge of diseases and their treatment. This may lead to poor compliance, withdrawal of therapy or inappropriate responses to adverse effects.

Some common problems of childhood (behaviour and sleep difficulties) are now considered by parents to be indications for drug therapy. This medicalization of aspects and variations of normal growth, behaviour and development, which may have resulted from biased media exposure or previous medical action, is reinforced by further inappropriate use of drugs.

Drugs

Suitable unit doses and formulations for children may not be available. Reliable information regarding efficacy and dosage from study data is still limited even for some commonly used drugs.

The prescriber

Many prescribers are poorly educated in the basic principles of prescribing for children.

Parents often exert inappropriate pressure on physicians to prescribe for their children even for mild, self-limiting conditions.

Overprescribing may result from excessive emphasis on the role of drug therapy in relation to other therapeutic approaches.

Doctors are under considerable pressure from drug companies to prescribe their products. The direct (interviews with sales representatives) and indirect (advertisements in medical journals) forms of this pressure may influence the prescriber to select less than optimal or greater than necessary therapy.

Most countries' health care systems by nature allow little time for consultation. This may increase the pressure to prescribe.

Drug response determinants

Rational drug therapy requires an understanding of the wide variability in drug handling and response that occurs in children, particularly in the first few years of life. Pharmacokinetics indicate what the body does to a drug, and pharmacodynamics, what the drug does to the body.

Pharmacokinetics

Absorption and bioavailability

Absorption is the passage of a drug from the site of administration through tissues or cell membranes to reach the blood. The rate and extent of gastrointestinal absorption of a drug depends on many factors, including the gastric emptying time, the acidity of the intestines, the presence of food, metabolism by the intestinal wall and microflora, and the effects of disease. After the neonatal period these factors change little, so with few exceptions gastrointestinal absorption varies little with age.

The rate of absorption, but not the extent, is increased by the use of liquid preparations, since no time for dissolution is needed. These are traditionally but not always appropriately prescribed for children.

Bioavailability is the percentage of the dose administered that reaches the systemic circulation. Metabolism by the intestinal wall or in the liver on first passage reduces the bioavailability of certain drugs such as propranolol, terbutaline and morphine, but this occurs in children in the same way as in adults.

The rate and extent of absorption from intramuscular sites and through the skin differs little according to age except during the period shortly after birth.

The lack of observed differences in drug absorption from infancy to adult life suggests that absorption changes little with age; the limited study data available confirm this.

Distribution

The main factors that influence distribution are the rate of absorption and rate of penetration of membrances, perfusion, the volume and

7

composition of tissue compartments, and the extent of binding to protein and tissues.

Some age-related differences in these factors are known. First the ratios of extracellular to intracellular water and total body water to body weight fall throughout childhood, most rapidly in the first 3 months. Body fat is low in the newborn, rises to a maximum at 9 months, then decreases until the age of 6 years. For the first few months of life the protein binding of most drugs is slightly lower than at other ages.

Organ perfusion varies more with disease than with age. Penetration of the blood-brain barrier is the same in infancy and childhood as in adult life.

Water-soluble drugs, which are distributed mainly in the extra-cellular fluid, have their largest relative volumes of distribution[a] in the neonatal period and early infancy, and these then decrease throughout childhood. The effects of age on the distribution of fat-soluble drugs are less predictable. For most drugs, plasma concentrations following a single weight-related dose and peak levels during continuous dosing are lowest during early infancy. The small differences in protein binding are not clinically important. For most drugs, therefore, the younger the child, the larger the weight-related dose required.

Biotransformation

Biotransformation is the process whereby drugs and their metabolites are made more water-soluble, thus enhancing their efficient excretion. Biological activity is not always reduced, as some drug metabolites are active.

The liver is the most important organ for biotransformation. The rate of metabolism depends on the size of the liver and the efficiency of hepatic enzyme systems, particularly the microsomal system, which is based mainly on cytochrome P450. These systems are responsible for oxidation, reduction and conjugation. Liver size may be less directly related in early infancy when some of its mass has a haemopoietic function. The ratio of liver volume to unit body weight decreases throughout childhood and is twice as great at 1 year as at 14 years. The metabolizing ability of liver tissue seems to be similar in children and adults, and the relatively large size of the liver in infancy is associated with more rapid oxidation, reduction and hydroxylation than at other ages. The clearance rates of many drugs decrease steadily throughout

---

[a] Volume of distribution is the conceptual fluid space into which a drug is distributed.

childhood. In the first few weeks of life, however, much drug metabolism is low, but increases rapidly from about 3 to 12 weeks.

Elimination

Because most drugs are eliminated through the kidneys, developmental changes that affect glomerular filtration and tubular secretion are the most important factors determining the rate and extent of elimination.

Surface-area-related values for glomerular filtration increase steadily in early infancy and reach adult values between 2.5 and 5 months of age. Thus, for instance, drugs that are primarily eliminated unchanged by the kidneys are eliminated slowly in the first months of life. Thereafter, elimination in childhood may be greater than in adults. Penicillins are also more slowly excreted until tubular secretion reaches adult values, after 2–3 months.

The factors affecting drug biotransformation and elimination have clear clinical implications. In early infancy, the clearance rates of drugs biotransformed in the liver and drugs excreted unchanged by the kidneys are low, and daily dose requirements are also low. After a few weeks of life, doses of drugs excreted by the kidneys increase and remain fairly stable throughout childhood, although the dose requirements of drugs that undergo biotransformation increase rapidly. Weight-related doses remain higher than for adults throughout most of childhood, gradually decreasing towards adolescence.

With repeated dosing at the usual intervals, the fluctuation of drug levels in the blood is least in early infancy but greatest in later infancy and early childhood. More frequent dosing is therefore needed throughout this period.

Individual variations in response

Children of similar age differ in their rates of drug biotransformation but show less marked differences in rates of elimination of those drugs primarily eliminated unchanged by the kidneys. These differences are probably due mainly to genetic factors, although disease and environmental and dietary factors may influence both rates, particularly the first.

Dose may have to be modified in children with hepatic and renal disease and specialist advice should be sought in such cases.

Pharmacodynamics

It is not known whether there are age-related differences in receptor sensitivity between children and adults. Receptor numbers and sensitivity

9

cannot yet be accurately determined *in vivo* and there is little available data relating pharmacological effect and plasma drug concentration. Children are reported to be more sensitive to parasympathomimetic agents but have higher tolerance of sympathomimetic drugs. Infants also require relatively higher doses of digoxin (as related to body weight or surface area), despite the fact that concentrations in the myocardium and the erythrocytes are comparatively high. A two- to three-fold increase in specific digoxin binding sites, as compared with adults, suggests a lower binding affinity in children.

In children paradoxical effects may occur with phenobarbital and amphetamines; amphetamines may reduce hyperactivity and children treated with phenobarbital may become more active, with difficult behaviour and a short attention span. Paradoxical stimulant effects may occur with sedatives, such as chloral hydrate and phenothiazines (such as alimemazine (trimeprazine) and promethazine); insomnia and irritability are the most common of these.

The prescribing process

Is a drug required?

This question may be difficult to answer, whether the drug is for specific treatment or for symptomatic relief. Drugs are often used in children for self-limiting conditions and for symptoms for which drug efficacy has not been established.

Problem areas include:

(*a*) antibacterial drugs used for upper respiratory tract infections that are usually viral;

(*b*) the overuse of decongestants for upper respiratory tract congestion, causing unacceptable adverse effects;

(*c*) the use of drugs in diarrhoea;

(*d*) the use of oral anti-emetics for vomiting;

(*e*) the use of antipyretic agents for fever;

(*f*) tricyclic antidepressant drugs used for nocturnal bed-wetting (these account for three quarters of deaths in children due to accidental poisoning);

(*g*) the sedation of sleepless children or those falsely labelled hyperactive;

(*h*) the use of spasmolytics in abdominal pain;

(*i*) the use of drugs to increase appetite; and

(*j*) the use of "prophylactic" immunoglobulins for small children with frequent upper respiratory tract infections.

In sum, these areas of drug use account for about 70% of all medicines taken by children, and therefore as much as two thirds of all drugs used by children may have little or no value. The medicalization of some presenting problems and the inappropriate use of drugs for other conditions may have important consequences for future prescribing in terms of parents' demand for and expectation of drug therapy. The psychological and social consequences for the child given drugs in

11

this way are not known, but children may tend to grow up believing that drugs are the solution to many of life's problems.

Choice of drug

There are seven considerations in drug selection.

Efficacy

This should have been established in clinical trials and/or practice in children. Where possible, it is preferable that new drugs be assessed in adults before children and in older children before newborn babies.

Low toxicity

Toxicity should be related to benefit as a risk/benefit ratio. In children, growth and development must always be considered, as adverse effects may not be immediately apparent. Growth delay due to systemic steroid use and staining of teeth by oral tetracyclines are important examples.

The therapeutic index, which indicates the difference between the toxic and effective concentrations of a drug, is generally similar in children and adults. Since there are fewer data on proper dosage for children, it is more difficult to be sure of staying between these limits. Where possible, one should choose another drug with a wider therapeutic index or monitor blood drug levels.

Clinical use and kinetic data availability

Clearly, it is better to use drugs for which full prescribing information is available, but even with detailed and comprehensive information, variability in children may prevent appropriate dosing in all cases.

Some drugs have been used for many years, yet information on their use in certain circumstances is still inadequate. These drugs include acetylsalicylic acid, paracetamol, tricyclic antidepressants, alimemazine, prochlorperazine and promethazine. Considerably more is known about some less commonly used drugs.

Cost

The clinician has a clear responsibility always to use the cheapest appropriate drug treatment.

Availability of an appropriate preparation

This is often a problem; for instance, children under 4 years are generally unable to use inhalers, so an alternative method of administration must be selected.

Risk of poisoning

The risk to the child or a young sibling from accidental ingestion must be assessed.

Combination products

The need to tailor drug doses to individual requirements in children generally precludes the use of inflexible fixed dose combinations. Those most widely used are cough suppressants, expectorants and systemic nasal decongestants, and all are of doubtful value.

Some preparations contain drugs with widely different kinetic profiles, and the rational use of one component is then impossible. This is a particular problem during maintenance dosing. Examples include fixed combinations of different anticonvulsants and of anticonvulsants with analgesic drugs.

The use of fixed combinations must be carefully monitored, as it may invoke a false sense of security arising from a questionable theoretical benefit. For example, children receiving thiazides with potassium salts or potassium-sparing agents may still become hypokalaemic. In addition, the large sizes of some of these preparations may make them more difficult for children to swallow.

The use of these preparations may have some advantages. Some are cheaper than the combined costs of their components, compliance may be improved by reducing the number of doses, the adverse effects of the omission of one or two vital drugs (as in tuberculosis therapy) may be prevented, and synergistic actions may be exploited.

Routes of administration and drug preparations

Oral route

This route is preferred for most children and most conditions, although vomiting often follows and may prevent absorption.

Tablets and capsules. Most children aged 4 years and over can swallow tablets of an average size, but many have difficulty with large capsules. Tablets can be crushed between two spoons and the powder mixed into a suitable drink or into food.

Most sustained-release formulations should not be cut, broken or crushed, but some capsules can be split and the contents emptied into a sugar-free liquid in the same way as crushed tablets.

Solid preparations, particularly those known to cause severe poisoning, should be stored in child-resistant containers or packages.

Labelling on containers should give as much information as possible, according to the guidelines in the section on information for children and parents (p. 31).

Children's preferences for certain colours and shapes do not affect compliance. It is dangerous for drug preparations to resemble sweets.

Liquid preparations. Liquid preparations are often but not always appropriately prescribed for young children; they have clear disadvantages. The shelf life is generally shorter than for solid preparations, particularly when dilution is used to increase the volume of a small dose to a standard 5 ml, and graduated spoons give inaccurate doses and allow spillage. In addition, many liquid medicines contain sucrose, particularly those sold over the counter. In chronic use these preparations can encourage bacterial plaque and gingival inflammation and lead to dental caries. The possibility that some preparations contain lactose must be considered when prescribing for children with lactose intolerance.

Some liquid medicines contain dyes and colouring agents such as tartrazine, to which sensitive children may react adversely. A few tablets also contain these agents.

Prescribers should therefore:

— prescribe tablets rather than liquids but, if this is not possible, prescribe liquids with sugar-free bases (if liquids containing sucrose have to be prescribed, a strict oral hygiene programme should be instituted during the treatment period);

— allow pharmacists to offer tablets rather than liquids; and

— advise parents of the risk of dental caries and encourage them to ask pharmacists for tablets rather than liquids.

Rectal route

Children dislike this route and it is in general unsatisfactory. It can seldom be relied on to provide predictable, adequate levels of drugs in the blood, and there may be a risk of toxicity due to erratic absorption (as in theophylline in aminophylline suppositories). It may, however, prove useful in the following circumstances.

14

Clonazepam and diazepam rectal solutions are rapidly and well absorbed and are effective in stopping convulsions. Absorption from suppositories is slower and their use is not advisable.

Anti-emetic suppositories offer an alternative to intramuscular injection to stop vomiting.

Rectal diazepam solution is effective in rapidly providing sedation for minor procedures.

Paracetamol suppositories may be used to reduce fever when the oral route is precluded.

Metronidazole suppositories can be used for pre-operative prophylaxis before bowel surgery.

Inhalation

Drugs for respiratory conditions, especially asthma, may be administered by inhalation. Sympathomimetic drugs are best given in this way as it achieves maximum benefit with minimum adverse effects. Cromoglicate disodium for preventing asthma can only be given by this route.

Children have difficulty in coordinating their breathing to inhale pressurized aerosols successfully, although modifications that act as reservoirs can be useful. Powdered preparations of such drugs as salbutamol and cromoglicate disodium are more likely than aerosols to be effectively administered, although children under 4 years of age seldom master this technique, either. Jet or ultrasonic nebulization may be used to deliver solutions of β_2-adrenergic stimulants, cromoglicate disodium, anticholinergic agents and steroids. This is the most efficient method of inhalation and children can use a mouthpiece or mask, according to preference.

Skin

Administration of drugs by topical application to the skin is usually appropriate only for skin conditions. Variable absorption may occur through inflamed or broken skin, and toxicity may occur from the widespread use of some preparations such as those containing steroids, boric acid and hexachlorophene when applied to areas of nappy rash.

Intramuscular

Injections into muscle are often painful and should therefore be avoided when possible; hydrocortisone, paraldehyde and erythromycin are particularly irritant. Further, intramuscular injection does not guarantee the systemic availability of all drugs. For instance, chloramphenicol and phenytoin are erratically absorbed and other drugs, such as digoxin, are no more quickly absorbed through this route than through oral administration. The drugs in many supposedly intramuscular injections are in fact deposited into subcutaneous fat, especially in older, obese children and adults. The quadriceps muscle is the recommended site for intramuscular injection. Examples of the use of intramuscular drug administration include:

— giving phenothiazines to stop vomiting, although the rectal route may also be used;

— using anticonvulsants to stop convulsions in children who have intercurrent illness with vomiting and who normally take non-parenteral drugs, such as sodium valproate and carbamazepine;

— using this route when treatment is essential and there has been failure of compliance; for instance, monthly injections of benza-thine benzylpenicillin are a useful alternative to oral phen-oxymethylpenicillin or pheneticillin in the prevention of rheu-matic fever (although this drug is not registered in all countries).

Dose size

Formulae have been devised to aid the calculation of dosage in children, but they are unsatisfactory. Most involve fractions of adult doses and take no account of the differences in kinetics and dynamics between children and adults. Their use is not recommended.

The following statements about children's doses are generally applicable.

— Drug doses related to surface area are similar throughout childhood.

— The younger the child, the larger will be the weight-related single dose of a drug; again, infants and younger children have larger volumes of distribution for most drugs.

— Total weight-related daily doses of drugs given long term, where these are mostly eliminated by the liver, will need to be highest in infants and much lower later on. As the child gets older the doses can gradually be reduced. In the first few weeks of life, daily doses are lower, since drugs are not cleared as well as at other ages, owing to hepatic immaturity (Fig. 3).

— Weight-related daily doses of drugs primarily eliminated by the kidneys are similar at most ages after about 6 months.

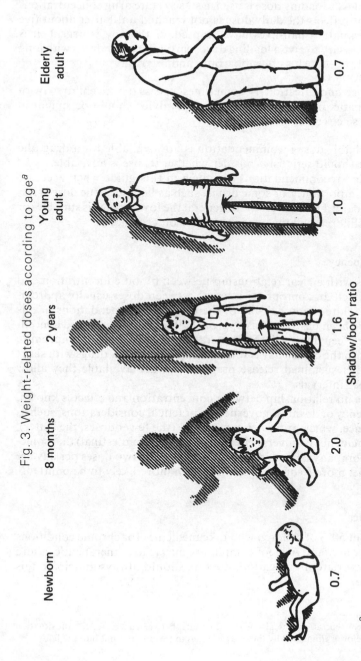

Fig. 3. Weight-related doses according to age[a]

Newborn	8 months	2 years	Young adult	Elderly adult
0.7	2.0	1.6	1.0	0.7

Shadow/body ratio

[a] The shadow indicates the dose relative to age, based on the young adult standard, for drugs eliminated mainly by the liver. The ratio of shadow to body size reflects the relative metabolic efficiency of the liver at each age.

17

— Unless a loading dose is used, a steady state drug concentration[a] that reflects the daily dose is not reached until after about five elimination half-lives have elapsed. If therapy is urgent, it is necessary to give a loading dose, particularly for drugs with long half-lives such as phenobarbital and digoxin.

— Dose modification is sometimes necessary in children with hepatic or renal disease. Specialist advice should be sought in these circumstances.

If a reliable dose recommendation is not available for a drug, the prescriber should seriously consider whether its use is advisable.

Detailed recommendations are given in this guide when accurate doses are important. For some drugs, such as laxatives, the dose is less important and a range is given. In general the lower range is suitable for younger children and the upper range for older children.

Dose frequency

For drugs with a clear relationship between blood concentration and clinical effect, an appropriate interval between doses usually approximates the elimination half-life of the drug. Recommendations in this guide have been based on this approach; fluctuations in blood concentration between doses will then generally be acceptable. A compromise to fit in with the child's day is sometimes necessary for drugs with short half-lives. If sustained release preparations are available they allow longer dose intervals.

Where no relationship between concentration and effect is known, the frequency of dosing is governed by practical considerations, such as convenience, which promotes compliance (the fewer doses, the better), and the incidence of adverse effects (mainly gastrointestinal) that sometimes accompany large doses. Generally, one or two doses per day are acceptable; more frequent doses are much more likely to be omitted.

Compliance

Only about 50% of children who take medicines for chronic conditions are fully compliant. As poor compliance may lead to therapeutic failure or inappropriate investigation, doctors should always anticipate this problem.

---

[a] The concentration that, although it fluctuates between doses, reflects the situation in which the drug eliminated by the body is equal to the amount put into the body.

18

The following steps would improve compliance.

— Prescribe the most appropriate medication, with full explanations of how it works, how to take it and for how long, how to store it, how it is expected to help and how to recognize problems that might arise. Written as well as verbal information should be given if possible.

— Plan and discuss the dose regimen at the start of therapy so that an unwritten "contract" is assumed. This should take account of periods of sleep, mealtimes, school hours and breaks, preferred formulations, easiest unit sizes, and rational and practical dose intervals based on kinetics. Decide at what times the drug should be taken, the best tablet size or volume of liquid, and whether the drug should be taken before, during or after meals. Note these things and explain them to the patient.

— Give medication as infrequently as possible. Choose the most palatable preparation possible. Give information on possible adverse effects, both the most likely and those that are rare but important. Open discussion should reduce the fear that may result in non-compliance.

Therapeutic drug monitoring

Facilities for the measurement of drug levels are not yet readily available to most physicians practising outside hospitals. The indications for monitoring levels are the same at all ages, but their clinical importance may be greater in children because:

— children vary widely in their handling of and responses to drugs;

— the margin of safety is often narrower than in adults; and

— the titration of dose to response is unreliable for many commonly used drugs, such as anticonvulsants.

Therapeutic drug monitoring is helpful in determining the doses most likely to provide effective and safe concentrations, in assessing compliance with therapy and in the interpretation and understanding of drug interactions. Blood sampling is the most appropriate approach and effective doses are determined by relating the concentration of drug in blood to the therapeutic range of the drug (the range of concentration within which maximum pharmacological effect is achieved in the majority of patients with minimum toxicity).

A knowledge of drug concentration without an appropriate interpretation of its significance is clinically useless. For maximum benefit, the prescriber needs to keep the following considerations in mind.

Duration of therapy

Unless a loading dose has been given, a steady state will not be reached until treatment has lasted for five elimination half-lives. Steady state levels should be measured after that time.

Dosing in relation to elimination half-life

The concentration of all drugs fluctuates, not necessarily to an acceptable degree, between doses, except when drugs are given by continuous infusion. Blood sampled immediately before dosing will generally reflect the lowest concentration in the dose interval. This may well be the best time to measure drug levels, although it is not always convenient, and samples taken at other times must be interpreted in the knowledge of the likely concentration time profile between doses. Signs of toxicity may occur when concentrations are at their peak and yet not be present at other times within the dose interval.

Active metabolites

Some drugs have active metabolites. These drugs include carbamazepine (10'11 epoxide) and primidone (phenobarbital and phenylethyl malonamide), and the pharmacological effects may be considerable and sometimes paramount. In such cases, measurement of the parent drug will be insufficient and concentrations of the metabolites require consideration.

Combination therapy

The possibility that one drug may affect the concentration (and therefore pharmacological effect) of another drug used in combination must always be considered (see p. 29).

Compliance

An undetectable drug concentration is easy to interpret as poor compliance or non-compliance. A lower concentration than expected is a more difficult problem and may lead to difficulties in recommending appropriate courses of action.

Remember that measuring and interpreting a child's plasma concentrations of drugs is only a small part of the information needed to treat a patient properly. It complements sound clinical judgement, but does not replace it.

Information about drugs for which therapeutic drug monitoring is useful, and in some cases necessary, to provide appropriate dosing advice is shown in Table 1. Drugs used almost exclusively in hospitals, such as chloramphenicol and aminoglycosides, have been excluded.

Table 1. Elimination half-lives, usual dose frequency and ranges of drugs for which therapeutic drug monitoring is indicated

Drug	Approximate half-life (h)	Usual dose frequency (times/day)	Therapeutic range mg/l (μmol/l) unless stated
Carbamazepine (remember 10'11 epoxide metabolite is active)	6–10	2–3	4–12 (16–50)
Digoxin	24–60	1–2	0.5–2.1 ng/ml (0.65–2.6 nmol/l)
Ethosuximide	30–40	1	40–100 (280–700)
Phenobarbital	30–40	1	10–35 (40–140)
Phenytoin	Varies with dose	2	10–20 (40–80)
Theophylline	3–5	2–3[a]	10–20 (55–110)

[a] Sustained release preparations should be used whenever possible; a prolonged absorption phase reduces fluctuation and allows less frequent dosing than that indicated by elimination half-life.

Drugs in breast-milk

Most drugs are excreted in breast-milk, but usually in amounts too small to harm the baby. Much advice on this subject has previously been based on single-case data. It is now clear that the problems have been overstated and many current recommendations are overcautious.

The concentration of a drug in milk usually but not always parallels that in plasma, and milk/plasma ratios for most drugs are between 1 : 3 and 1 : 1. The total amount available for absorption by the infant is generally small, less than 2% of the total maternal dose.

Some infants in the first weeks of life, such as pre-term and jaundiced babies, are at greater than normal potential risk. The risk decreases as renal and hepatic function improve with increasing age. Infants with glucose-6-phosphate dehydrogenase (G-6-PD) deficiency and those with an allergic tendency are also at increased risk from some drugs, although these conditions are seldom evident at the time.

Idiosyncratic reactions, unrelated to dose or concentration, may theoretically occur in spite of the low milk concentrations, but this is very seldom of clinical importance.

Approach to drug therapy

Although the risk for most drugs is negligible, the prescriber should generally be cautious. If drugs are necessary, a suitable preparation can almost always be found. Single-dose treatment does not represent a risk.

Mothers who must have treatment should not be prevented from breastfeeding unless there is information to suggest that the drug is unsafe. The few contraindicated drugs include those used in cancer chemotherapy (cytotoxics), ergot alkaloids and radiopharmaceutical agents. A safe alternative drug is generally available. The least potentially toxic drug compatible with the appropriate treatment of the mother should be used.

Information and guidance should be available from a paediatrician or pharmacologist with special interest in this problem or from a drug information centre. The likely drug concentration in breast-milk and thus the daily dose for a baby on an average milk intake can be calculated. A direct assay of the drug concentration in milk may be helpful in checking predicted amounts.

The infant's condition should also be closely monitored. Some effects are predictable. These include bradycardia and hypoglycaemia with beta-blockers (β-adrenergic blocking drugs), anticholinergic symptoms with atropine, or sedation with psychotropic drugs.

Finally, where appropriate, the baby's blood levels and other related functions, such as blood film/count and thyroid function, should be checked.

Although this approach is relevant to all drugs that might harm the baby, it is particularly important for those drugs for which a theoretical risk exists. These include anticoagulants, antithyroid drugs, atropine, beta-blockers, bromocriptine, chloramphenicol, clemastine, diazoxide, diuretics, gold salts, H_2-receptor antagonists, isoniazid, lithium, oral hypoglycaemics, nalidixic acid, narcotics, nonsteroidal anti-inflammatory agents and oral steroids. These drugs are seldom given to breastfeeding mothers, however, and we are not aware that problems have resulted in practice from their use.

For some drug groups the use of one drug is preferred to that of another, such as propylthiouracil rather than carbimazole, and warfarin rather than phenindione.

Adverse effects

Apart from the elderly, drugs have adverse effects most frequently on newborn babies. Theoretically, infants and children might be more at risk than adults because of their variations in drug handling and response.

If doctors told families more clearly about the potential problems of drug therapy, adverse effects would be more readily recognized and reported by parents and then by doctors. The efficacy of a system for reporting adverse effects would depend on such early reports from physicians, including mention of cases in which the causal connection is not proven.

When adverse effects are suspected, a precise drug history is essential and must include non-prescribed drugs administered by parents. These account for almost half of the drugs taken by children in many countries. Most adverse effects occur in the first week or two of therapy. The most powerful diagnostic tool is rechallenge (giving the drug again), but this may be dangerous and should only be done when specifically indicated, as in cases in which the drug is likely to be required again for a life-threatening condition. It should then be given only under carefully controlled conditions, usually in hospital.

Specific adverse effects

Adverse drug reactions may be related to dose (concentration-related). If they are not related to dose (idiosyncratic), they often have an allergic basis and occur at each exposure to the medication; they are also less likely to be reversible.

Some drugs have specific adverse effects on growth and development. For example, tetracyclines stain the teeth, cytotoxics cause fertility and growth problems, and systemic corticosteroids retard growth. These drugs should not be used in children if there is an alternative. Further, children may react paradoxically to drugs affecting the central nervous system (phenothiazines, amphetamines, sympathomimetics and chloral hydrate) and have a greater tendency to dyskinetic reactions with metoclopramide and phenothiazines. Some adverse effects may be prevented by measurement of drug levels (see p. 21) but the most important factors are rational prescribing and continued vigilance by the prescribing physician.

Certain adverse effects occur in children with specific disorders; haemolysis may occur in children with G-6-PD deficiency when exposed to some drugs. The drugs that are reported to cause haemolysis and that have been considered in this book are listed below.

analgesics	acetylsalicylic acid
antimalarials	chloroquine
	primaquine
nitrofurans	nitrofurantoin
sulfonamides	mafenide
	sulfamethoxazole
sulfones	dapsone
miscellaneous	chloramphenicol
	vitamin C

Some adverse effects may occur some years after drug use. For example, diethylstilbestrol given to women in high dosage during pregnancy resulted in vaginal carcinoma in their offspring 20 or more years later. Data on drug prescription should therefore be retained for at least 25 years.

Interactions

Drugs may interfere with the action of other drugs used concurrently. The frequency of interactions is directly related to the number of drugs prescribed. Long lists of potential interactions have been published, but few have clinical relevance.

Generally, the mechanisms and effects found in children are similar to those in adults, but many of the drugs more commonly implicated are seldom used in children, such as oral hypoglycaemics and warfarin, and children more often take only one drug.

Problem drugs

Anticonvulsants, such as carbamazepine, phenobarbital and phenytoin, induce hepatic enzymes; they may thus reduce the concentration of other drugs metabolized by the liver and impair their effects. For example, when phenobarbital is used to prevent convulsions in meningitis, serum chloramphenicol concentrations may be reduced to inactive levels; when enzyme-inducing anticonvulsants are given with oral contraceptives there is a risk of pregnancy. Rifampicin has a similar effect on hepatic enzymes.

Cimetidine, isoniazid and chloramphenicol are enzyme inhibitors and so may increase the concentration of drugs metabolized by the liver and increase their effects.

Phenobarbital elixir contains alcohol and can produce disulfiram reactions with other drugs, such as metronidazole and latamoxef.

Erythromycin inhibits theophylline metabolism and so increases its concentration and effect.

Finally, sodium valproate displaces phenytoin from binding sites and so temporarily increases its effect.

Therapeutic drug monitoring can be important in defining and monitoring the interaction of drugs, especially anticonvulsants.

Information for children and parents

Children and their parents need to be informed in order to use medicines safely and effectively. The doctor is clearly responsible for giving appropriate information. This should be done in full and open discussion with the parents and the child about the proposed treatment. As in other aspects of management, the prescriber should form a cooperative alliance with the family, and together they should plan the best and most convenient way of managing the problem. In most cases this will involve discussion about non-drug alternatives to usually accepted therapies. These may include changes in diet, behavioural treatment and physiotherapy, which may replace or complement the other approaches.

The following check list may help to provide clear and specific information. Written information cannot, however, be tailored to cover every individual, or replace oral information from the physician. An information sheet, similar to that shown in Table 2, may be used.

What children and parents need to know

1. The name of the medicine.

2. The reason for using it.

3. When and how to take it.

4. How to know if it is working effectively, and what to do if it is not.

5. What to do if one or more doses are missed.

6. The risks of omitting medication.

7. How long to continue taking it.

8. The most likely side effects, those that are unlikely but important, and what to do if they occur.

9. Whether other medicines can be taken at the same time.

10. The alternatives to drug therapy.

31

Table 2. Information sheet

Drug management	Information needed
How the drug is to be taken	Dose per formulation and number of units Suggested clock time (to be agreed) Time between doses Time before or after food Duration of treatment
Storage of the drug	Container Type of cupboard Temperature Expiry date Signs of deterioration
How the drug is expected to help	Symptoms Consequences of good or bad compliance Time to achieve effect Signs of effect Action to take if no effect
Recognizing problems due to the drug	Signs Action to take

Poisoning

Children may be poisoned accidentally by drugs, chemicals and poisonous plants, and poisoning is a common indication for admission to hospital.

A poisoning accident may be caused by:

— a child's exploratory activity, particularly in children aged 18–36 months;

— doctors' prescription of excessive doses of drugs or mistakes by pharmacies;

— a child mistaking drugs for sweets;

— inadequate or inappropriate drug storage or supervision;

— adolescent suicide attempts or cries for help; or

— (rarely) the inappropriate administration of drugs by parent(s), as a form of abuse or overzealous treatment.

Poisoning could in large part be prevented if all drug suppliers used child-resistant containers or packaging and if all dangerous products were correctly used and stored. It is important that all drugs can be identified by name on the packaging. In many countries legislation to establish these practices has greatly reduced the incidence of poisoning, which is fortunately no longer an important cause of mortality.

The possibility of poisoning should be considered in the diagnosis of acute illness in childhood, particularly when unusual or unexpected symptoms are present. The most important feature in the diagnostic approach is to get a thorough medical history. This is in general the basis for further diagnostic and therapeutic intervention.

Diagnostic approach

When a clear history of drug ingestion cannot be obtained, the diagnostic approach should include:

— obtaining information about the drugs stored at home or taken by any of the household members;

— smelling the breath to detect solvents, and inspecting the lips and mouth for burns (caustic chemicals), discoloration and parts of tablets;

— examining vomitus, which may allow tablet identification, and retaining a sample of vomitus where possible; and

— looking for signs and symptoms that may suggest the causative agent, such as hyperventilation from salicylates; respiratory depression from barbiturates; fever, dilated pupils, dry mouth and tachycardia from atropine; or oculogyric crises and dyskinesia from phenothiazines or metoclopramide.

Immediate management

1.   Examine the child. Assess the child's general condition, particularly the level of consciousness.

2.   Secure the airway and resuscitate as necessary.

3.   Obtain a history, including where possible the name of the drug and the amount and time of ingestion.

4.   Obtain the container and label if possible; remember, this may not be an absolute guide as the contents may have been transferred from another container.

5.   Empty the stomach unless the patient is comatose or convulsing, more than two hours have elapsed since ingestion (or six hours for acetylsalicylic acid), or the poisoning is due to corrosives or petroleum products. Give 15 ml (5 ml for children under 1 year) ipecacuanha paediatric emetic (total alkaloids, as emetine, 14 mg/10 ml) followed by at least 200 ml of juice or water. It is more rapidly effective if the child is asked to run and move around or is bounced up and down on someone's knee. This can be repeated after 20 minutes if no vomiting has occurred. Remember that milk, apart from increasing the gastric absorption of petroleum distillates and lipid-soluble products, retards the emetic effect of ipecacuanha.

6.   Activated charcoal (50 g) may be useful in reducing the absorption of a number of drugs and may be particularly useful in tricyclic poisoning. Rapid ingestion may cause vomiting. The place of activated charcoal as compared with emesis or gastric lavage is still uncertain.

7.   Give antidotes or take other specific measures in the few circumstances where appropriate (Table 3).

Table 3. Antidotes for poison

Drug	Antidote
Disinfectants	milk, liberal fluids
Iron	deferoxamine (lavage using 2 g/l water; leave 10 g in 50 ml in the stomach)
Morphine and analogues (such as diphenoxylate)	naloxone 400 μg (1 ml) intravenously and 400 μg (1 ml) intramuscularly (may be repeated every 2–3 minutes to a maximum of 2.5 mg)
Organophosphorus insecticides	atropine, pralidoxime mesylate (at a hospital)
Paracetamol	acetylcysteine (at a hospital)
Phenothiazines } Metoclopramide }	procyclidine hydrochloride, intramuscularly or intravenously <1 year: 2.5 mg 1–4 years: 2.5–5 mg 5–12 years: 5 mg or biperiden 0.04 mg/kg; may be repeated every 30 minutes (maximum 4 doses)

8.   Contact a poisons information unit or centre to check that all appropriate measures have been taken.

To refer or not to refer to hospital

A decision can usually be based on the history and the presence or absence of symptoms. Children should always be referred to hospital when significant amounts of the following substances have been or may have been ingested:

acetylsalicylic acid	paracetamol
atropine	quinidine
digoxin	tricyclic antidepressants
diphenoxylate plus atropine	sustained release preparations
ergotamine	other toxic chemicals,
iron	corrosives and petroleum products

Children may not need to be admitted if other drugs have been taken, sufficient time for absorption has elapsed, and if:

— they have no symptoms;

— a family doctor is informed;

— the parents can be trusted to contact a doctor or hospital if symptoms develop; and

— delayed problems are not expected.

The gastrointestinal system

Antacids

Indications for use

Dyspeptic symptoms are uncommon in children, and these drugs are used mainly for symptomatic relief in gastro-oesophageal reflux and to promote healing in oesophagitis and peptic ulcers.

Prescribing guidelines

Aluminium hydroxide and magnesium trisilicate liquid preparations are as effective as most available proprietary preparations and are the drugs of choice.

For gastro-oesophageal reflux, give after meals when symptoms are most intense.

Higher doses, given frequently, are required to promote the healing of ulcers.

Useful drugs

Aluminium hydroxide is probably preferable to magnesium trisilicate, which often causes diarrhoea.

For hiatus hernia and gastro-oesophageal reflux, give 5–15 ml aluminium hydroxide within 30 minutes of completing meals. For peptic ulcer and gastritis, give 15–20 ml every 2–3 hours between meals and at bedtime.

Anti-emetics

Nausea and vomiting in children, especially babies, can be symptoms of a wide variety of underlying disorders. The determination of the underlying cause and appropriate management are important. Treating the symptom of vomiting may delay diagnosis.

Most vomiting in childhood will respond to treatment of the underlying disorder, and anti-emetic therapy is not usually required.

Indications for use

These are:

— migraine

— motion sickness

— cytotoxic therapy

— post-operatively, usually to counteract the effect of opiates.

Prescribing guidelines

Give only for specific indications.

Anti-emetics given by mouth may be of benefit in treating nausea, but once vomiting has started, use the rectal or parenteral routes. If vomiting can be anticipated, then oral prophylactic treatment may be effective.

Therapy needs to be given only while symptoms persist.

Most effective anti-emetics have considerable adverse effects, including sedation, dystonic reactions and anticholinergic effects. Their benefits must therefore be weighed against them.

Vomiting associated with cytotoxic chemotherapy may be anticipated by both prescriber and patient; a dose of an anxiolytic agent on the day before chemotherapy may prevent it.

Vomiting will stop once the underlying problem has been treated.

Alternatives to drugs

Simple reassurance or relaxation therapy may be valuable alternatives to drugs. Psychotherapy may also be tried in complicated cases.

Useful drugs

The drugs of choice are antihistamines, specifically the H_1-receptor antagonists.

Piperazine group

Drugs of this type, such as cyclizine and cinnarizine, are useful mainly in preventing motion sickness, although they are less effective than hyoscine.

All piperazines are sedative, but generally their adverse effects in pharmacologically effective doses are less than those of hyoscine and they are better tolerated.

They differ in the onset and duration of their effect, but not in their efficacy. (Cinnarizine has the slowest onset.)

	Dosage per day		Route	Timing of first dose
	1–4 years	5–12 years		
cyclizine		25 mg three times	oral	30 minutes before journey
cinnarizine	7.5 mg three times	7.5–15 mg three times	oral	2 hours before journey
dimenhydrinate	25 mg three times	35 mg four times	oral or rectal	30 minutes before journey

Phenothiazine group

These drugs are not effective in motion sickness, but may be useful for vomiting associated with migraine (note that migraine is often associated with slow gastric emptying, see p. 100), cytotoxic therapy and in the post-operative period.

Prochlorperazine and perphenazine are less sedating than chlorpromazine, but dystonic reactions are seen equally with all. These reactions are not dose-related and are relatively common. Procyclidine or biperiden rapidly stops these effects (see p. 35).

39

	Form		Dose	
			1–4 years	*5–12 years*
prochlorperazine	oral {	acute attack	5 mg initially then 2.5–5 mg after 2 h	10 mg initially then 5 mg after 2 h
		prevention	2.5 mg twice daily	5 mg twice or three times daily
	deep intramuscular injection		3.125–6.25 mg as required; do not repeat within 6 h	6.25–12.5 mg as required; do not repeat within 6 h
	rectal		5 mg twice daily	5 mg three times daily

The adverse effects of prochlorperazine include drowsiness, dry mouth, dizziness and extrapyramidal dystonic reactions.

Hyoscine

This is effective for preventing motion sickness. Drowsiness, dry mouth, dizziness and blurred vision are adverse effects, but are not common at the following oral dose given once only:

Age	*Dose*
1–4 years	75–100 μg
5–12 years	100–300 μg

Metoclopramide

This drug has similar anti-emetic activity to phenothiazines, but probably is slightly less potent. Its activation of peripheral motility in the gastrointestinal tract, as well as its central anti-emetic action (chemoreceptor trigger zone and vomiting centre) may make it more useful in vomiting due to gastrointestinal and biliary disease.

Metoclopramide is particularly useful in vomiting associated with cytotoxic therapy and the first dose should be given before therapy begins.

Age	*Oral dose*	*Intravenous dose*
<1 year	1 mg twice daily	2 mg/kg every 2 h up to a maximum of 10 mg/kg in 24 h
1–4 years	2 mg twice or three times daily	
5–12 years	2.5–5 mg three times daily	

Adverse effects include extrapyramidal effects (see p. 35).

Domperidone

This may be useful for children receiving cytotoxic therapy, but should probably only be used when other drugs have failed. It is available only for oral or rectal use.

Spasmolytics

Indications for use

The use of these drugs in childhood is extremely limited. Few children have peptic ulcer, typical irritable bowel syndrome or diverticular disease, the main indications for their use.

Prescribing guidelines

There is little convincing evidence that children who scream with updrawing of the legs (often considered to be due to intestinal colic) respond better when anticholinergic drugs are administered than when full explanation and support alone are offered to parents. One of these drugs, dicycloverine, has been widely prescribed, but it is no longer recommended for this indication as some instances of respiratory depression have occurred.

Useful drugs

Metoclopramide

This drug is useful in the treatment of heartburn, reflux oesophagitis and hiatus hernia, and more particularly as an anti-emetic (see section on anti-emetics, p. 38).

For reflux oesophagitis and hiatus hernia the dose is:

Age	Dose
<1 year	1 mg twice daily
1–2 years	1 mg twice or three times daily
3–4 years	2 mg twice or three times daily
5–12 years	2.5–5 mg twice or three times daily

Extrapyramidal adverse effects are more common in children than in adults.

Antidiarrhoeal drugs

Indications for use

Diarrhoea may be a symptom of infection, organic disease requiring investigation, or drug therapy (most commonly by antibiotic alteration of bowel flora). Infection may be due to bacteria, protozoa or more frequently viruses such as *Rotavirus*. It is not possible to differentiate clinically between viral and bacterial gastroenteritis. *Campylobacter* spp., *Salmonella* spp., *Shigella* spp. and enteropathogenic or enterotoxigenic strains of *Escherichia coli* are the most frequent bacterial causes. It is now known that oral glucose/electrolyte solutions are well absorbed even in diarrhoeal illness, so oral rehydration is appropriate in all but the most severe degrees of dehydration.

Diarrhoea may be spurious when there is faecal impaction with overflow.

Prescribing guidelines and alternatives to drug therapy

Determine the underlying cause if possible.

In infants and children, most cases are infective, and the first thing to do is to prevent or treat fluid and electrolyte depletion or imbalance. If there are signs of moderate or severe dehydration, hospital care is indicated. Most young children can be managed by removing solids and milk from their diet and giving them frequent small volumes of appropriate fluid and electrolyte mixtures. Home-made solutions containing table salt and sugar, if made up with a special spoon or other accurate measure, may be appropriate, but these contain no bicarbonate or potassium and their continued use after 48 hours is inadvisable. Parents' ability to understand instructions varies and there is also a real risk that errors in composition may arise. Excessive salt content in particular may be dangerous. A special or proprietary formulation containing these salts in appropriate proportions should be used instead. "Resting" the bowel for 24 hours, reintroducing milk at increasing strengths ($\frac{1}{4}$, $\frac{1}{2}$, $\frac{3}{4}$) in 12-hourly stages and gradually reintroducing solids usually proves satisfactory.

Some children aged 1 year and over seem to want more than just clear fluid. Some formulations are made up in acceptable fruit flavours and small amounts of flavouring added to the fluid mixtures may increase acceptance.

The oral replacement fluid recommended by WHO contains 20.0 g glucose, 3.5 g sodium chloride, 1.5 g potassium chloride and 2.5 g sodium bicarbonate per litre. The recommended sodium concentration is the maximum, and lower concentrations may be appropriate.

Antidiarrhoeal drugs have a limited role in the treatment of diarrhoea and should not be used in children under 2 years of age. They may be used if diarrhoea continues for more than 48 hours or in children over 6 years of age, but generally only as an adjunct to other approaches. Adsorbent mixtures are used for the relief of symptoms but are probably of little value.

Spasmolytics are not generally effective for diarrhoea, have unpleasant side effects and should not be used.

Antibacterial agents have no place unless a specific organism, for which treatment is indicated, has been isolated. They prolong the carriage of bacterial enteropathogens.

Diarrhoea that does not abate within four or five days should be investigated by laboratory examination and the culture of faeces. Malabsorption syndrome and persistant disaccharide intolerance should be considered.

Useful drugs

Paediatric kaolin mixture

This is an adsorbent mixture that should be given in the following dosage:

Age	Dose
1–4 years	10 ml every 4 h
5–12 years	15 ml every 4 h

Loperamide

Drugs that reduce gut motility have a place in the symptomatic treatment of chronic diarrhoeas such as Crohn's disease. Loperamide is more effective and safer than diphenoxylate as it does not enter the central nervous system and cause sedation. Diphenoxylate is therefore obsolete. Loperamide comes in 2-mg capsules or as an elixir (1 mg/5 ml).

	Age	Dose
loperamide	1–4 years	1 mg twice or three times daily
	5–8 years	1 mg four times daily
	9–12 years	2 mg four times daily

Persistent diarrhoea, particularly when associated with weight loss, requires investigation, although in healthy, thriving young children, investigation and treatment are usually not required.

Laxatives

Constipation is a common problem for children, but may be both underdiagnosed and overdiagnosed as many parents have misconceptions about normal bowel habits and press their doctors to respond to variations in normal patterns.

Indications for use

Laxatives should be used for:

— acquired megacolon, which usually presents as faecal retention with overflow
— pain
— impaction
— clearance of the bowel for surgery, radiological and endoscopic procedures
— prophylaxis in children known to have painful anal fissures.

Prescribing guidelines

Dietary approaches should be tried initially; laxatives can often be avoided in infants and children.

Stimulant laxatives may cause more pain than the problem for which they are used.

Laxatives are often required for children with mental and physical handicap and children regularly receiving narcotic analgesics.

Dry hard stools require softening agents in addition to laxatives.

Enemas or suppositories should be used if stools are impacted.

Avoid phenolphthalein which may cause rashes or albuminuria.

Alternatives to drugs

Possible alternatives to drugs are:

— to increase fluid intake; children often drink relatively small amounts per day;

45

— to increase natural lubricants, such as olive oil or prune juice, in the diet; or

— to increase fibre in diet by providing more fruit, wholemeal bread, bran cereal and vegetables, although it is difficult to change family eating habits.

Useful preparations

Bulking agents

These increase faecal mass and stimulate peristalsis. They may cause obstruction if adequate fluid intake is not maintained. Unprocessed bran is cheap, but even in orange juice or sprinkled on food it is unpalatable for many children. Ispaghul husk is an alternative but not much more palatable. Although some proprietary fibre preparations are tasteless, these are expensive.

Bran should be given in a dose of 5–15 g per day (in divided or single dose). Use the lower end of the dose range for younger children. Some proprietary cereals have a high bran content and are palatable to most children.

Osmotic agents

Lactulose, a semi-synthetic disaccharide, produces an osmotic diarrhoea by drawing water from the intestinal wall. The starting dose in the form of elixir (3.5 g/5 ml) should be:

Age	Dose	
<1 year	2.5 ml	
1–4 years	5 ml	twice daily
5–12 years	10 ml	
>12 years	15 ml	

The dose may be increased until the desired effect is achieved.

Faecal softeners

Docusate sodium is a detergent that mixes with and softens faeces, and this may cause enough rectal stimulation to increase bowel action.

Form	Dose	
Syrup	12.5–25 mg (5–10 ml)	three times daily
Tablets	20 mg	

Liquid paraffin should not be used. It causes anal leakage and irritation. Inhalation into the lungs producing a lipid pneumonia is a particular problem in children who do not cooperate fully with administration.

Stimulant laxatives

These all increase motility, but may cause abdominal cramp.

bisacodyl	tablets rectal solutions suppositories	2.5–7 mg at bedtime according to response
senna (= sennoside B)	tablets (7.5 mg) syrup (7.5 mg/5 ml) granules (14.9 mg/5 ml)	5–20 mg at bedtime 5–10 ml at bedtime

Rectal preparations

Suppositories may be be necessary in faecal impaction, but if these are ineffective enemas should be used. Some parents find the insertion of suppositories distasteful. Gloves should be provided.

Bisacodyl or glycerol suppositories are available, the latter in various sizes for different ages.

Arachis oil and various phosphate enemas can be used, although the latter should not be used for more than three days.

Appetite stimulants

Many parents have inappropriately excessive expectations about the food requirements of their children. They need a full explanation and reassurance; their children eat quite normally in most cases.

True anorexia is often psychogenic but may have an organic cause that should be identified. Appropriate therapy may then be indicated. There is no scientific evidence that the drugs and mixtures that are proposed as appetite stimulants have any effect on appetite. Therefore these preparations should not be used.

Ulcer-healing drugs

Peptic ulcers are uncommon in children. They may respond to treatment with antacids, but specific healing drugs may be required. These are also indicated in reflux oesophagitis.

Cimetidine and ranitidine reduce gastric acid output by H_2-receptor blockade. They should only be used in confirmed cases of ulcer or oesophagitis, and then only under the supervision of a specialist.

The cardiovascular system

Cardiac glycosides
and cardioactive agents

Cardiac failure and arrhythmias are rare in infancy and childhood compared with their frequency in adults. It is therefore generally advisable to seek specialist opinion before therapy is instituted.

Cardiogenic shock is unlikely to present to primary care doctors as it arises mainly in the early newborn period or in the first few hours after cardiac surgery. It will not be discussed here.

Supraventricular tachycardia (SVT) is the most frequent form of tachycardia and should be suspected in any infant with a heart rate of 200/min or more. Ventricular tachycardia is rare. Both forms of tachycardia are indications that specialist advice should be sought, and therapy should not be started at home except in emergency. In all cases an electrocardiogram is vital.

Vagal stimulation by carotid sinus massage, Valsalva manoeuvre or covering the nose with a cold cloth may cause reversion of SVT to normal rhythm.

Indications for use

In congestive cardiac failure, specialist opinion and advice should be sought before drug therapy is started.

With SVT, infants usually present in cardiac failure, particularly if SVT has been present for more than 24 hours. There is often an underlying Wolff-Parkinson-White syndrome or other conduction defect. Specific diagnosis and investigation are urgently required, and only then should therapy be given. Intravenous or orally administered digoxin usually produces reversion to sinus rhythm if given in an emergency. Digoxin is still the drug of first choice for maintenance therapy and prophylaxis. Direct current shock under specialist supervision is indicated in intractable tachycardias. In occasional conduction defects digoxin may be contraindicated.

Prescribing guidelines

Specific diagnosis and specialist advice should always precede therapy.

Useful drugs

Digoxin

This is the most commonly used glycoside. The elimination half-life (20–60 h) allows its use once daily, although local gastrointestinal effects may be reduced if a smaller dose is given twice daily. The maintenance dose is 5–15 μg/kg each day in one or two doses.

Precautionary note: digoxin is extremely dangerous in overdosage. The dosage should always be carefully checked; the elixir (50 μg/ml) is prescribed with a graduated pipette to simplify dosing.

Symptoms and signs of adverse effects vary with age. For example, the newborn may not "feed so well"; in infants, vomiting follows anorexia and diarrhoea, unlike in adults when vomiting comes first; toddlers, in addition to anorexia and diarrhoea, have drowsiness, headache, tingling in the hands and feet, and a feeling of "sadness".

Arrhythmias and electrocardiogram abnormalities can occur at all ages. Bradyarrhythmias occur more often than tachyarrhythmias, and marked bradycardia and heartblock are the most common problems.

If digoxin toxicity is suspected, the drug should be be discontinued and the child referred for specialist advice.

It may be helpful to measure the plasma digoxin concentration (the therapeutic range is 0.5–2.1 ng/ml (0.65–2.6 nmol/l); see p. 23).

Diuretics

Children generally handle and respond to diuretics in a similar way to adults. In most countries, children's diets provide sufficient potassium to compensate for the potassium lost in diuretic therapy.

Indications for use

These are:

— cardiac failure

— oedema and ascites, e.g. nephrotic syndrome

— hypertension, although this often responds poorly to diuretics alone and other drugs are usually required.

Alternatives to drugs

Restriction of salt in cooking and at the table is important to prevent fluid retention in nephrotic syndrome. It may also help and hasten the effect of diuretics in hypertensive children. A diet of saltless food sometimes causes children to stop eating, however, and this is counter-productive as protein intake is reduced. In some cases it may be better to allow salt and then to remove it by the use of diuretics.

Prescribing guidelines

The choice and route of administration of the drug is determined by the urgency of action or the severity of the oedema. In acute heart failure, potent loop diuretics with rapid action, such as furosemide and eta-crynic acid, are indicated; for long-term therapy, less intense and longer acting drugs, such as thiazides, are more suitable, particularly in older children.

Dosing should be in the mornings to avoid disturbing sleep in older children.

Additional potassium is required only if cardiac glycosides (digoxin) are used with potassium-losing diuretics. In such cases and if practical, potassium supplements (but not bicarbonate salts) should be given out of phase with diuretic dose times, e.g. diuretic in the morning, potassium supplement in the evening. An alternative approach is to give diuretics on four days per week with a three-day rest. The plasma potassium should periodically be measured.

These drugs should not be given to potentially hypovolaemic children with nephrotic syndrome without first expanding the plasma volume with "salt-poor" albumin, and then only under specialist supervision.

There is no advantage in using combined thiazide and potassium preparations unless there is a compliance problem.

Useful drugs

Loop diuretics

Furosemide acts within 30 minutes of oral administration. The effect lasts for up to 6 hours and is longest in infancy before the glomerular filtration rate has reached adult surface area related values (< 7 months).

The normal dose of furosemide is 1–3 mg/kg each day orally, but it may need to be increased to 5 mg/kg in severe heart failure. The use of divided doses may then be indicated. Special paediatric formulations are available, but sometimes the intravenous preparation used orally is more convenient, for instance in the young infant. Efficacy is judged by urine output and weight loss.

The adverse effects of furosemide are deafness, which may occasionally occur when high doses are used with aminoglycosides, potassium loss, diarrhoea, nausea and metabolic alkalosis.

Etacrynic acid and bumetanide are similar in effect to furosemide, but there are no established specific dosage guidelines.

Thiazides

Thiazides take longer to act and last longer (12–24 h) than loop diuretics. A number are available and all have much the same effect. Commonly used thiazide diuretics are bendroflumethiazide and hydrochlorothiazide.

	Daily dose
bendroflumethiazide	250–500 μg/kg on alternate days
hydrochlorothiazide	1–4 mg/kg (in one or two divided doses)

The adverse effects of thiazides are hypokalaemia, rashes and thrombocytopenia.

52

Potassium-sparing drugs

Spironolactone is a competitive aldosterone blocker and potentiates loop and thiazide diuretic action. Potassium supplements are not required and should not be used. The dose is 3 mg/kg each day in one or two divided doses for all ages.

Triamterene is an aldosterone antagonist. The dose is 2–4 mg/kg each day in one or two divided doses.

Osmotic diuretics

These include mannitol. They have no place in the home management of children. In hospital, they are used mainly to reduce intracranial pressure.

Anti-arrhythmic drugs

These drugs are infrequently required in children. They should only be administered under specialist supervision. The most common arrhythmia is supraventricular tachycardia, but only in infants does this generally persist long enough to cause cardiac failure (more than 24 hours).

Supraventricular tachycardia should be suspected in any infant or child who presents with a heart rate above 200/min. For maintenance and prophylactic therapy digoxin, sometimes combined with other drugs, remains the drug of first choice.

Ventricular tachycardias are rare and usually serious. Urgent specialist treatment is necessary to avert death.

Antihypertensive drugs

Primary hypertension occurs in children and is probably greatly under-recognized, since blood pressure measurement is unfortunately seldom included in the routine examination of children. The assessment of the need for therapy, and if so its management, is a specialist matter.

Respiratory tract disorders

The upper respiratory tract is the most frequent site of infection in children. The large majority of such infections are viral in origin. Antibiotics are not indicated unless there is a strong suspicion that bacteria are implicated. Symptomatic treatment, e.g. with antipyretics and analgesics, can be of considerable benefit. Decongestants and cough suppressants are often used but of doubtful benefit. The following sections discuss the use of these drugs and also include a consideration of management approaches for common upper respiratory tract problems.

Antipyretics/analgesics

The commonly used drugs have both antipyretic and analgesic actions.

Indications for use

Fever is an indication when symptomatic or where there is a recent, previous or family history of febrile convulsions.

Note that liability to febrile convulsions decreases rapidly after the age of 3 years.

Established pain is also an indication, as is the prevention of pain during anticipated painful procedures.

Prescribing guidelines

Pain and fever usually have an underlying cause, and this should be elicited. If it is amenable to treatment, e.g. otitis media, appropriate therapy should be given.

Once a treatable cause of either pain or fever has been excluded, symptomatic treatment can be given.

The treatment of pain is obviously to relieve distress, but the treatment of fever is to make the patient feel more comfortable and, in certain instances, to reduce the risk of convulsions associated with an elevated temperature.

In some cases fever has no symptoms, and antipyretics may therefore be unnecessary. It may also be counterproductive if it decreases the signs of disease, if it encourages the use of drugs for self-limiting mild disease, and possibly if it modifies a beneficial physiological response to infection.

Simple analgesics are satisfactory in most cases, but stronger analgesia, including opiates, may sometimes be required, e.g. after trauma or surgery.

Always use child-resistant packages.

Useful drugs

Paracetamol

This is the preferred drug for the prophylaxis and management of fever. It has fewer adverse effects than acetylsalicylic acid and is just as effective.

To reduce and prevent fever in children who have previously had febrile seizures, paracetamol should be given repeatedly every 4 hours, following a loading dose. If the night-time dose is omitted the next (morning) dose should be larger in order to "load" again.

Loading (first) dose: 10–15 mg/kg for all ages

Subsequent four-hourly doses: 7–12 mg/kg for all ages

If the night dose is omitted, next dose: 10–15 mg/kg for all ages

For general pain relief and to reduce fever which is symptomatic, it should be given as required but not more often than every 4 hours, in an oral dose of 7–12 mg/kg.

The same dose may be given rectally as suppositories or as a liquid drug by using a syringe or rectal tube dispensers.

Adverse effects are uncommon but an overdose may cause hepatic toxicity.

Acetylsalicylic acid

This should be avoided in children under 1 year (saturation kinetics appear to be responsible for greater toxicity at this age) and probably also in older children as there is some evidence that acetylsalicylic acid may be one factor in causing Reye's syndrome, a dangerous encephalopathic disease of childhood. It may be necessary, however, to use it in children with juvenile chronic arthritis.

Age	Oral dose	
1–4 years	75–225 mg	each dose up to four-hourly,
5–12 years	300–450 mg	preferably after food

Note that fluid intake should always be encouraged in febrile children.

For the adverse effects of acetylsalicylic acid see p. 155.

Additional antipyretic measures

Remove the child's clothes during episodes of fever. Cool with a fan or tepid sponging/bathing, though this carries the danger that core temperature may be unaffected or rise. Both methods should be used in conjunction with drugs. Cooling with alcohol or cold baths should be discouraged. It is important to give full instructions on the management of subsequent fevers to the parents of a child who has had a febrile convulsion.

Cough suppressants

Cough suppressants are potentially dangerous as they may cause sputum retention. They should not be used if the cough is productive. They may have some value when dry cough prevents the child and his family from sleeping at night.

If a cough is persistent or recurrent, consider the possibility that the child has pertussis, foreign bodies or underlying asthma (see section on anti-asthma drugs, p. 63).

Drugs

The drugs available are all in linctus form. Relatively cheap examples are: noscapine linctus, linctus codeine and linctus codeine paediatric. Linctus codeine is very potent in relation to childhood dosages: inadvertent overdosage may easily result.

	Age	Dose	
linctus codeine paediatric (codeine phosphate 3 mg/5 ml)	< 1 year 1–4 years	5 ml 10 ml }	up to five times daily
linctus codeine (codeine phosphate 15 mg/5 ml)	5–12 years	5–10 ml	up to five times daily
noscapine linctus (1 mg/ml and 2.5 mg/ml)	1–4 years 5–12 years	5–10 mg 10–15 mg }	up to three times daily
dextromethorphan (tablets 15 mg, liquid 15 mg/ml)	< 1 year 1–4 years 5–11 years	2.5 mg 7.5 mg 10 mg }	up to four times daily

Expectorants and mucolytics

Although these drugs are widely prescribed, there is no evidence that they are more effective than placebo preparations. They usually include subemetic doses of ammonium chloride, ipecacuanha or squill. Many contain several pharmacological ingredients, often illogically including a cough suppressant. The use of these preparations is irrational and inappropriate.

Although the use of simple expectorants as placebos is preferable to inappropriate antibiotic prescription, this practice is not to be recommended. If such an approach is followed, a simple cheap preparation should be used, such as ammonia and ipecacuanha mixture, in a dose of 2.5–10 ml up to four times daily according to age. The claimed effectiveness of mucolytic agents remains to be demonstrated (see p. 78).

Decongestants

Nasal obstruction can be very distressing to the young child and may make feeding difficult. Mucosal oedema may also block the eustachian tube and lead to painful distension of the eardrum.

Indications for use

These are:

— significant nasal obstruction, particularly in a baby or toddler in whom feeding may be affected; and

— distension of the tympanic membrane.

Prescribing guidelines

Decongestants can be given topically or systemically. Nasal irrigation with 0.9% saline is safe, effective and cheap, and may be useful in young children. All decongestants have α-adrenergic effects and may cause hypertension and behavioural effects in overdose. There is no evidence that preparations that contain anti-infective or antihistaminic agents are more effective.

Useful drugs

Topical decongestants

These include oxymetazoline (0.025% and 0.05%) and xylometazoline hydrochloride (0.1%) which are both effective for 8–12 hours. The dose should be according to the duration of action (1–3 drops or two applications of spray for all ages). Use the lowest concentration in babies under 1 year. All topical decongestants can be given as nasal drops or sprays. The method of instillation of nasal drops is important: the child should lie flat and fully extend his neck.

All topical decongestants can produce rebound vasodilation and increased nasal obstruction with continued use. Tachycardia may also occur. Treatment should not be continued for more than a few days.

Systemic decongestants

They may cause hallucinations and behavioural effects in some children. They are of no proven benefit.

Drugs for upper respiratory tract allergy

An allergic etiology should be considered if upper respiratory tract symptoms are persistent or seasonal. Although antihistamines may be helpful, mast cell stabilizers and topical steroids have fewer side effects and are more likely to be of benefit.

Indications for use

These are:

— hay fever/pollinosis

— allergic rhinitis/sinusitis.

Prescribing guidelines

Cromoglicate disodium or a topical steroid are the treatments of choice. The first-line approach is cromoglicate disodium by nasal drops or spray prophylactically, although it has to be given so often (six times per day) that it may prove impractical.

If symptoms persist, topical steroids can be applied either on their own or in combination with systemic antihistamines, although those in current use often produce unacceptable sedation in children.

For occasional short-term acute problems, such as critical school examinations, systemic steroids may be given.

Desensitizing injections may be dangerous and probably have little place in the management of children with upper respiratory tract allergy.

Useful drugs

Mast cell stabilizers

Cromoglicate disodium is available as a spray and as nose drops, which either on their own or in combination with antihistamines often control nasal allergy. The dose is 20 mg three or four times daily for all ages.

61

Topical steroids

These are inhaled. Several preparations are available: beclometasone, flunisolide, budesonide, betamethasone and tixocortol.

Antihistamines

There is now a large number of antihistamines available; they differ in their sedative action, duration of effect and adverse effects.

All have the potential to produce sedation, headache and anticholinergic effects, including dry mouth, blurred vision and gastrointestinal dysfunction such as constipation.

Some newer antihistamines, such as terfenadine, are considered to have less sedative effect, but their place in the management of this condition remains to be established.

Alternatives to drugs

Hyposensitizing injections

Desensitizing courses should be given only after carefully evaluating the severity of the child's symptoms while on an adequate trial of conventional therapy and when a clearly proven allergic cause is present. The discomfort and potential risk of this form of treatment (anaphylaxis, angio-oedema and allergic rashes) must be considered. The risks may be greater in children than in adults. The effect of injections is uncertain. There is unlikely to be any benefit if there is an allergy to more than one allergen, which is usually the case.

Arrange to start the course of desensitizing injections early enough to complete the course before exposure to the antigen is likely to occur: for pollens, for instance, start in January. Give the injections at one- or two-week intervals with increasing strength over about ten weeks. Commercially available sets contain three to five strengths, e.g. Alavac-P, Allpyral-G, Norisen Grass and Spectralgen Pollens (Single Species). Injections should be given only where resuscitation equipment and trained personnel are available. Observe the child for 60 minutes after the injection. Do not give further injections if any severe allergic reaction occurs.

Drugs for the treatment of asthma

A diagnosis of asthma should be considered in any child who has recurrent attacks of wheeze or cough.

Indications for use

Asthma is common: 5–12% of children are affected. It is often undiagnosed and may be under-treated even after diagnosis.

Although respiratory tract infections are common precipitants of asthma attacks, bacterial infection is uncommon and antibiotics are not usually indicated. Anxiety in the child is a rare precipitant but frequent accompaniment of asthma. Effective bronchodilator therapy usually relieves anxiety, and there is little place, if any, for the use of anxiolytics and sedatives. The house dust mite, a commonly implicated allergen, cannot practically be eliminated from or significantly reduced in homes.

Prescribing guidelines

Drug therapy is the most effective treatment for asthma but it can be complex and delivery is difficult in young children. As in many other therapies, it is most important to give a full explanation (which may include written information) to both child and parents.

Drug therapy may be ineffective if the administration technique is faulty. Proper teaching, regular demonstration and checking will reduce these problems.

Drug therapy

Drug therapy is sometimes descriptively subdivided into prophylactic and bronchodilator groups. Cromoglicate disodium and inhaled steroid preparations are considered to be prophylactic agents, and β_2-adrenergic stimulants, intravenous aminophylline and oral or intravenous steroids to be bronchodilator drugs. In fact, most (but not cromoglicate disodium) may be considered to fulfil both roles, as is the case for theophylline preparations.

63

An approach to drug therapy for the newly diagnosed asthmatic child is outlined in the flow diagram in Fig. 4. It may be considered to represent an inverted ladder with each increasing section or rung indicating a more intensive approach. Some countries in Europe have a different approach and use theophylline at an earlier stage.

An approach to the therapeutic management of the child with an acute asthmatic attack is outlined in a similar way in Fig. 5.

Useful drugs

β_2-adrenergic stimulants

These are safe and highly effective. Parents and children should be encouraged to use drugs early, rather than wait until symptoms have been present for some time. By that stage, mucosal oedema and intraluminal secretions will be contributing to airways obstruction.

Most β_2-adrenergic stimulants can be given either orally or by inhalation. The oral route is simple and the effect generally lasts longer, but it has the disadvantage that considerably more of the drug reaches the systemic circulation and produces adverse effects: tremor, jumpiness and tachycardia (in spite of relatively selective β_2 stimulation).

With inhalation the effect is felt more rapidly (in 1–3 min) than with the oral route (in 15–45 min), there is a greater degree of bronchodilation, better prevention of exercise-induced bronchoconstriction, and a much smaller dose is necessary.

The aerosol technique is critical, and if there is any doubt about a child's ability to use a device, an alternative system should be used. Although children differ in their ability to use inhaling devices, the following guidelines are suggested for effective therapy.

Age	Capacity
< 1 year	Cannot usually inhale efficiently through any device
1–2 years	Can usually inhale from nebulizer/compressor system
2–4.5 years	Some proprietary inhalers, e.g. Nebuhaler, Spacers and do-it-yourself devices such as coffee cup reservoir/aerosol combinations, can be used effectively by some but not all children
4.5–10 years	The above methods and powder inhalation devices such as the rotahaler and the spinhaler, are usually effective. The direct use of aerosols is ineffective in many children
> 10 years	Most children can use aerosol inhalers directly as well as the above methods

There is little evidence that any one preparation is preferable, but some, particularly salbutamol and terbutaline, are available in a variety of formulations and delivery devices and are therefore more flexible. Salbutamol and terbutaline are also available in sugar-free formulations.

The inhalation dose is many times smaller than the oral dose, and many suggested dosages are very conservative. For salbutamol or an equivalent preparation, it is safe to use up to two puffs $(200\mu g)$ for 1–4-year-olds and up to three puffs $(300\mu g)$ for 5–12-year-olds, up to 10 times a day, provided the child's condition is not deteriorating (suggested by inability to speak sentences, "pulsus paradoxus", severe tachycardia or tachypnoea, or any degree of cyanosis).

β_2-adrenergic stimulants are usually not effective in the first 15 months of life.

Older nonselective sympathomimetic drugs, e.g. epinephrine, isoprenaline and orciprenaline, should no longer be used as they have more adverse effects and a short duration of action, the latter applying particularly to epinephrine and isoprenaline.

The β_2-adrenergic stimulant drugs that are commonly available are shown in Table 4.

Cromoglicate disodium

This is a prophylactic drug which is remarkably free of adverse effects. It has no effect on the relief of acute attacks and may irritate the airway and exacerbate the attack at that time. It must be taken by inhalation, usually 3–4 times daily.

Form	Dose
pressurized aerosol (1 mg/puff)	two puffs 3–4 times daily
powder inhalation of Spincaps (20 mg per capsule) using a Spinhaler or Halermatic insufflator	20 mg four times daily
respirator solution (10 mg/ml)	20 mg four times daily

The powder formulation is also available in combination with isoprenaline sulfate, but this combination is not recommended.

For children under 5 years, the respirator solution is generally most effective, although some 4-year-olds and occasionally some 3-year-olds can take the powdered formulation efficiently.

During coughing and wheezing attacks, a β_2-adrenergic stimulant respirator solution can be added to the cromoglicate disodium solution.

Therapy may not appear to be effective for some weeks, and a trial of therapy should last for at least three months.

Fig. 4. Long-term management of asthma

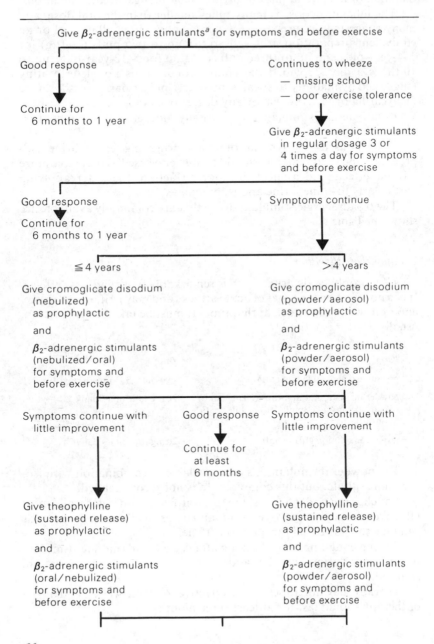

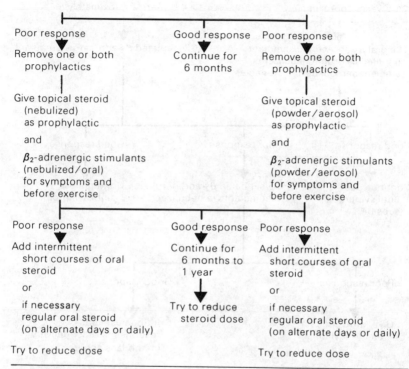

Poor response
Remove one or both
  prophylactics

Give topical steroid
  (nebulized)
  as prophylactic

and

β_2-adrenergic stimulants
  (nebulized/oral)
  for symptoms and
  before exercise

Good response
Continue for
6 months

Poor response
Remove one or both
  prophylactics

Give topical steroid
  (powder/aerosol)
  as prophylactic

and

β_2-adrenergic stimulants
  (powder/aerosol)
  for symptoms and
  before exercise

Poor response
Add intermittent
  short courses of oral
  steroid

or

if necessary
regular oral steroid
  (on alternate days or daily)

Try to reduce dose

Good response
Continue for
6 months to
1 year

Try to reduce
steroid dose

Poor response
Add intermittent
  short courses of oral
  steroid

or

if necessary
regular oral steroid
  (on alternate days or daily)

Try to reduce dose

[a] Drugs should be given orally or by proprietary "reservoir" inhalers to children aged 4 years and under. They should be inhaled in powder/aerosol form by children over 4 years of age. Jet nebulizer can be used by either age group. Drugs should be taken to treat symptoms and for prophylaxis before exercise.

Fig. 5. Management of the acute asthma attack

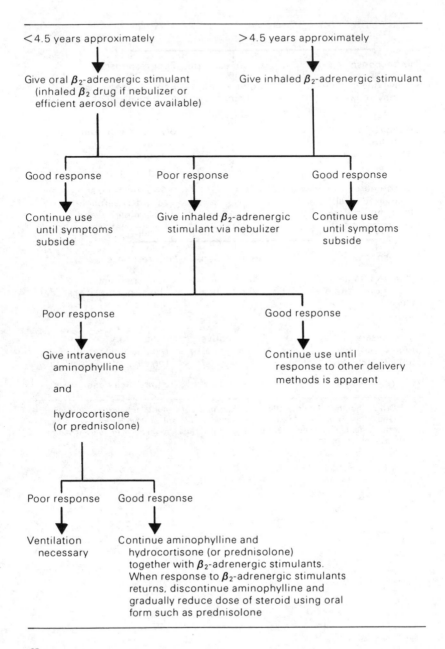

<4.5 years approximately

Give oral β_2-adrenergic stimulant
(inhaled β_2 drug if nebulizer or
efficient aerosol device available)

>4.5 years approximately

Give inhaled β_2-adrenergic stimulant

Good response

Continue use
until symptoms
subside

Poor response

Give inhaled β_2-adrenergic
stimulant via nebulizer

Good response

Continue use
until symptoms
subside

Poor response

Give intravenous
aminophylline

and

hydrocortisone
(or prednisolone)

Good response

Continue use until
response to other delivery
methods is apparent

Poor response

Ventilation
necessary

Good response

Continue aminophylline and
hydrocortisone (or prednisolone)
together with β_2-adrenergic stimulants.
When response to β_2-adrenergic stimulants
returns, discontinue aminophylline and
gradually reduce dose of steroid using oral
form such as prednisolone

Xanthine derivatives

Theophylline and aminophylline are rapidly eliminated from the body. The half-life of theophylline in children is 3–5 hours. With most oral formulations absorption is rapid and, unless they are given about every 4 hours, large fluctuations in plasma concentrations occur between doses. This is important as the bronchodilator effect is related to plasma concentration. A therapeutic concentration range of 10–20 mg/l (55–110 μmol/l) is established for adults (see p. 23) and is probably valid for children, although lower concentrations may be effective.

Adverse effects include headache, anorexia, diarrhoea, nausea, vomiting, tachycardia, palpitations, insomnia, arrhythmias, convulsions and even death, all of which may occur with increasing concentrations above 20 mg/l. The narrow therapeutic range limits their clinical value, and the use of traditional preparations such as choline theophyllinate, diprophylline and etamiphyllin is not recommended. However, there are now sustained-release preparations that prolong absorption and reduce the fluctuation between usual dose intervals, allowing administration twice daily in most children over 7 years. Doses should be given three times daily for most children under 5 years.

Because there is a wide variability of drug handling in children, plasma levels of theophylline should be measured when these drugs are used.

A scheme for starting and maintaining theophylline therapy is shown in Fig. 6.

Xanthine derivatives come in a variety of forms.

Oral. A number of sustained-release preparations are available. Most are large and children under 3 years have difficulty swallowing them. Some are in capsule form containing pellets and these can be administered without the capsule. They may be spread on food or given in spoonsful of sucrose-free liquids. Some preparations have better sustained-release properties than others.

Intravenous. Aminophylline is effective in severe asthma by slow (over 15 min) injection of 5 mg/kg, but except in acute emergency this should be given in hospital only. Note that if the child is receiving chronic theophylline therapy — always ask about this — the use of aminophylline by injection for acute attacks is not recommended unless drug levels and heart rhythm (by electrocardiogram) are monitored and full resuscitation facilities are available.

Table 4. β_2-adrenergic stimulants

Drug	Form
Fenoterol	Aerosol (180 μg per puff) Respirator solution (50 μg/ml) (dilute 4–20 times)
Pirbuterol	Elixir (7.5 mg/5 ml) Capsule (10 mg) Aerosol (200 μg per puff)
Reproterol	Elixir (10 mg/5 ml) Tablets (20 mg) Aerosol (500 μg per puff) Respirator solution (100 μg/ml) (dilute 4 times)
Rimiterol	Aerosol (200 μg per puff) Auto aerosol (200 μg per puff) Respirator solution (500 μg/ml) (dilute 2 times)
Salbutamol	Elixir (2 mg/5 ml) Tablets (2 mg and 4 mg) Sustained-release tablets (8 mg) Aerosol (100 μg per puff) Inhaler powder (200–400 μg) Respirator solution (100 μg/ml) (nebules) Intravenous/intramuscular injection (50 μg/ml)
Terbutaline	Elixir (1.5 mg/5 ml) Tablets (2.5 mg and 5 mg) and sustained-release tablets (5 mg and 7.5 mg) Aerosol (250 μg per puff) Aerosol spacer (250 μg per puff) Respirator solution (2.5 mg/ml) Intravenous/intramuscular injection (500 μg/ml)

[a] β_2-adrenergic stimulants are usually not effective in the first 15 months of life.

[b] Dose given for special inhalation devices.

Dose			Suggested maximum number of doses per day (see also text)
1 year[a]	1-4 years[b]	5-12 years	
—	1-2 puffs	1-3 puffs	Up to 10
500 µg	500 µg-1.0 mg	500 µg-1.5 mg	Up to 10
3.75 mg	3.75 mg	7.5 mg	Up to 4
—	—	10 mg	Up to 4
—	1-2 puffs	1-3 puffs	Up to 10
5 mg	5 mg	10 mg	Up to 4
—	10 mg	10 mg	Up to 4
—	1-2 puffs	1-2 puffs	Up to 10
2.5 mg	5 mg	5-10 mg	Up to 6
—	1-2 puffs	1-3 puffs	Up to 10
—	—	1-3 puffs	Up to 10
6.25 mg	6.25 mg	6.25-12.5 mg	Up to 6
2 mg	2 mg	2-4 mg	Up to 4
—	2 mg	2-4 mg	Up to 4
—	—	8 mg	Single dose
—	1-2 puffs	1-3 puffs }	Up to 10
—	200 µg	200-400 µg }	
2.5 mg	2.5 mg	2.5-5 mg	Up to 6
—	4-6 µg/kg		Single dose
0.75 mg	1.5 mg	1.5-3 mg	Up to 4
—	2-5 mg	2.5-5 mg	Up to 4
—	1-2 puffs	1-3 puffs	Up to 10
—	1-2 puffs	1-3 puffs	Up to 10
—	1.25 mg	1.25-2.5 mg	Up to 6
—	10 µg/kg		

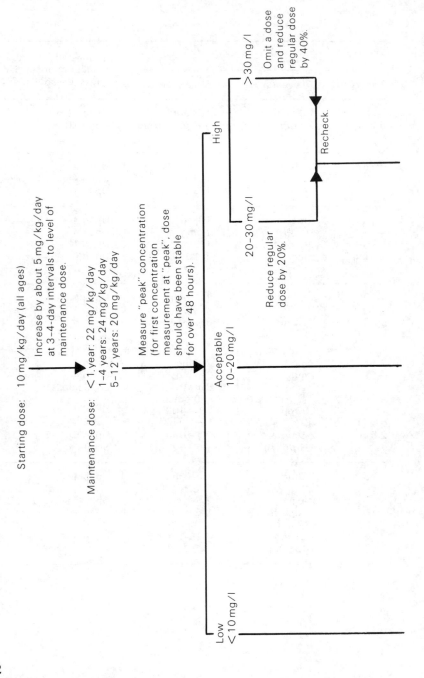

Fig. 6. Scheme for starting and maintaining theophylline therapy in chronic asthma

Starting dose: 10 mg/kg/day (all ages)

Increase by about 5 mg/kg/day at 3–4-day intervals to level of maintenance dose.

Maintenance dose: < 1. year: 22 mg/kg/day
1–4 years: 24 mg/kg/day
5–12 years: 20 mg/kg/day

Measure "peak" concentration (for first concentration measurement at "peak", dose should have been stable for over 48 hours).

Low
< 10 mg/l

Acceptable
10–20 mg/l

High

20–30 mg/l

Reduce regular dose by 20%.

> 30 mg/l

Omit a dose and reduce regular dose by 40%.

Recheck.

72

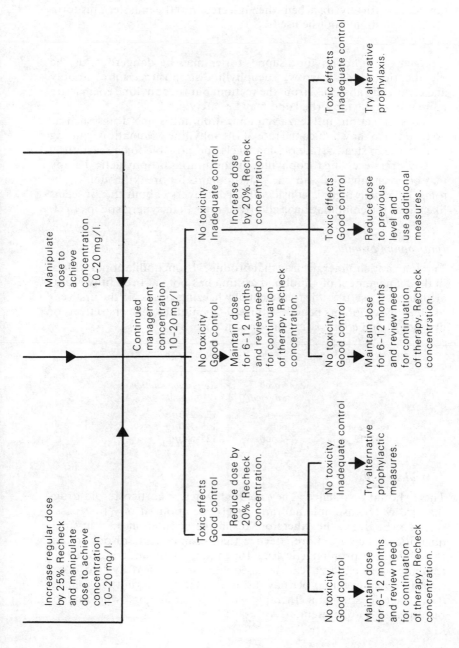

Increase regular dose by 25%. Recheck and manipulate dose to achieve concentration 10–20 mg/l.

Manipulate dose to achieve concentration 10–20 mg/l.

Continued management concentration 10–20 mg/l

Toxic effects
Good control

Reduce dose by 20%. Recheck concentration.

No toxicity
Good control

Maintain dose for 6–12 months and review need for continuation of therapy. Recheck concentration.

No toxicity
Inadequate control

Try alternative prophylactic measures.

No toxicity
Good control

Maintain dose for 6–12 months and review need for continuation of therapy. Recheck concentration.

No toxicity
Good control

Maintain dose for 6–12 months and review need for continuation of therapy. Recheck concentration.

No toxicity
Inadequate control

Increase dose by 20%. Recheck concentration.

Toxic effects
Good control

Reduce dose to previous level and use additional measures.

Toxic effects
Inadequate control

Try alternative prophylaxis.

73

Intramuscular. Aminophylline and theophylline are painful, irritant and erratically absorbed when injected into the muscle. This form of injection should not be used.

Rectal. Aminophylline suppositories may be dangerous, as the therapeutic index is narrow. Theophylline suppositories are variably and erratically absorbed from the rectum, but theophylline enemas are more predictably absorbed and may be safely used.

Virus infection, influenza immunization and some drugs such as erythromycin may reduce the rate of theophylline elimination, causing an increase in steady-state plasma levels and possible toxic reactions.

Children receiving theophylline as continuous prophylactic therapy may be given inhaled β_2-adrenergic stimulants for breakthrough symptoms. Although there is considerable controversy about this, it seems likely that the combination is additive rather than synergistic in effect.

Ipratropium bromide

This is an anticholinergic drug that produces bronchodilation. Its place in the management of childhood asthma has not yet been fully evaluated, but it is useful in the treatment of wheezing attacks in the first year of life; 40% of infants benefit within 10–20 minutes. Adverse effects of dry mouth and constipation are uncommon.

Age	Dose (every 3–4 h)	
	Aerosol (18μg/puff)	*Respirator solution (250μg/ml)*
<1 year	—	125–250μg
1–4 years	1 puff	125–500μg
5–12 years	1–2 puffs	125–500μg

Topical steroids

These should be inhaled. They are highly active corticosteroid drugs that are water-insoluble and are largely metabolized on "first pass" through the liver. They therefore reach the circulation only in small quantities. They are more effective than cromoglicate disodium and theophylline as prophylactic drugs for children with moderate to severe asthma. Most children can be adequately controlled by two doses (morning and evening) per day, using regular or intermittent inhaled β_2-adrenergic stimulant therapy whenever coughing, wheezing or breathlessness are present.

Their adverse effects include oral thrush (in 2–5%) which can be treated with antifungal lozenges (p. 116) without discontinuing therapy. Dysphonia can also occur. In large doses, such as over 1600 μg per day of beclometasone, some systemic side effects may occur, including excessive weight gain and even cushingoid appearance. The pituitary–adrenal axis may also be suppressed but its clinical significance is uncertain.

There is no evidence that any one preparation is more effective than the others in clinical practice. Examples of commonly used drugs are the following.

— Beclometasone comes in the most forms and therefore has the greatest flexibility in use. It is the only one available as a nebulizer suspension, but as yet the effectiveness of this preparation is unproved by controlled trials.

— Betamethasone is more potent than beclometasone.

— Budesonide lasts slightly longer, and can be given by the Nebuhaler or Spacer inhaler.

Dose frequency	Form	Dose		
		< 1 year	1–4 years	5–12 years
beclometasone 2–4 times daily	respirator suspension (50 μg/ml)	50–100 μg	50–200 μg	—
	inhaled powder (100 μg and 200 μg)	—	100–200 μg	100–400 μg
	aerosol (50 μg and 250 μg/puff)	—	—	50–250 μg
betamethasone 2–4 times daily	aerosol (100 μg/puff)	—	—	100–300 μg
budesonide twice daily	aerosol (50 μg and 200 μg/puff)	—	50–200 μg[a]	50–200 μg

Systemic steroids

These are indicated for various forms of severe asthma. For severe acute asthma which has not responded to inhaled β_2-adrenergic stimulants or to intravenous aminophylline, the dose is 100–200 mg intravenous hydrocortisone every 4 hours for all ages or oral prednisolone 1–3 mg/kg each day in 2–3 doses. The response may be delayed for 6–8 hours. When the response to inhaled or injected β_2-adrenergic

---

[a] Can be given by the Nebuhaler.

stimulants is regained, then oral steroids such as prednisolone can be started in those children who were given intravenous hydrocortisone in the dose shown above, or continued for a short course in those already given prednisolone, either stopping the therapy or weaning off it within 2–7 days.

For several severe acute attacks leading to hospital admission, consider providing the parents with courses of prednisolone in appropriate dosage to give to their child, so that they can begin this therapy as soon as the child begins to deteriorate.

In severe asthma that cannot be controlled with inhaled steroids, with regular inhaled β_2-adrenergic stimulants by nebulizer or with sustained-release theophylline, then use prednisolone. The dose is 1–2 mg/kg each day, reducing to one 5–10-mg dose on alternate days as soon as possible (see p. 133).

Continue to give all children topical steroids and regular β_2-adrenergic stimulants to keep the systemic steroid dose to a minimum. Alternate day dosage is preferred, but some children are not controlled on the day off.

For the adverse effects see the section on corticosteroids, p. 133.

Alternatives to drugs

Desensitization

Controlled trials report that the benefit of desensitization is limited to a small reduction in conventional drug therapy. This small benefit should be weighed against the need for long courses of injections and the risk of local or systemic reaction. Desensitization should only be given to children who have severe symptoms that are difficult to control with the currently available standard therapy and who can be demonstrated to have a severe reaction to one particular allergen, e.g. house dust mite.

Elimination of house dust mites

Attempts to reduce the number of house dust mites are almost always unsuccessful. Traditional approaches, such as damp dusting and frequent vacuum cleaning, are therefore probably useless in the management of asthma.

Hypnosis, acupuncture, humidifiers, changes in climate

Each of these forms of therapy has advocates, but there have been no controlled trials that have shown their benefit.

Admission to hospital

Any one of the following is an urgent indication that the child should be admitted to hospital:

— cyanosis

— drowsiness/semi-coma

— respiratory distress with no improvement after two doses of inhaled β_2-adrenergic stimulants one hour apart

— acute attack in a child who previously needed ventilation.

Exercise-induced bronchoconstriction (EIB)

Drug therapy

Prevention or improvement by prophylaxis is the preferred approach. The timing and frequency of therapy depend on the onset and duration of drug activity.

First-line approach. β_2-adrenergic stimulants such as salbutamol (200 μg by inhalation) are 90–100% effective. They take effect immediately or within 5 minutes. Dose immediately before or during exercise. The effect will last 2–6 hours. Drugs that are inhaled are much more effective than those taken orally.

Second-line approach. Cromoglicate disodium (20 mg) is effective in 70–80% of children. The optimal time for therapy is 30 minutes before exercise. The effect lasts 2–4 hours.

Third-line approach. A combination of the above drugs should be given.

Alternative or complementary approaches

Nasal breathing reduces EIB. For training programmes, artificial warming and humidifying masks can be used as warm, humid air reduces EIB. A careful choice of activities can limit EIB. Short burst sports and swimming produce the least EIB and water polo, American football, baseball, cricket and circuit training are all recommended.

Drugs for the treatment of cystic fibrosis

Regular physiotherapy, to assist in the expectoration of sputum, is essential in the management of cystic fibrosis.

Useful drugs

Four groups of drugs are used regularly in the management of cystic fibrosis. Two are related to the lung problems (antibiotics and mucolytic agents) and two to the gastrointestinal tract (pancreatic enzymes and vitamin supplements).

Antibiotics

In an acute exacerbation, any antibiotic chosen should work against *Staphylococcus aureus* and *Haemophilus influenzae* but it should be selected on the results of sputum culture and sensitivity tests whenever possible. Antibiotics must be given in higher than usual dosage to be effective.

Some authorities keep children up to 1 year of age on continuous antistaphylococcal therapy using flucloxacillin or cloxacillin. Later other organisms, particularly *Pseudomonas* spp., *Proteus* spp. and *Klebsiella* spp., become a problem, and intravenous courses of aminoglycosides (such as gentamicin and tobramycin) combined with antipseudomonal penicillins (such as carbenicillin, piperacillin and azlocillin) and appropriate cephalosporins are indicated. Some paediatricians prescribe antibiotics to be given by inhalation, using a nebulizer and compressor at home, but there is little evidence that this is an effective approach.

Mucolytic agents

Mucolytics have been used widely in the hope that they might reduce viscosity and allow the child to cough up sputum more readily. There is little evidence that the inhaled preparations such as acetylcysteine (20% solution) have any short-term or long-term advantages over inhaled steam and physiotherapy alone.

Pancreatic enzymes

Most children with cystic fibrosis have malabsorption and require pancreatic enzyme supplements. In the young child these can be taken as powders mixed with liquids or feeds, at the beginning of each meal. For older children tablets or granules are preferable. Capsules are also available that can be taken whole or emptied on to the food immediately before eating. There are many preparations available and these vary widely from country to country. The dose should be titrated against the stool consistency to ensure that the child thrives and that steatorrhoea is minimized. Sodium supplements are indicated for some children in warm climates.

The adverse effects of pancreatic enzyme supplements include irritation of the skin around the mouth and anus. Siblings or parents may occasionally have allergic reactions to the powder formulations.

Some children continue to suffer from steatorrhoea, in spite of the use of pancreatic supplements in high dosage and acid protective formulations, e.g. enteric-coated preparations. Increasing the gastric, duodenal and jejunal pH by the use of an H_2-receptor antagonist will reduce enzyme inactivation and bile salt precipitation, and therefore steatorrhoea. An improvement in fat absorption will ensue.

Vitamin supplements

These are required by all children and the fat-soluble vitamins are particularly important.

The central nervous system

Psychotropic drug use in children is only appropriate when no reasonable alternative is available. These drugs powerfully influence brain function, and this last-line approach to drug therapy is particularly important in children since little is known about the effects of these drugs on the development of brain function.

Overuse, which is common, may result from or lead to the usually inappropriate conclusion that a child's problems are medical rather than behavioural or social.

Indications and prescribing guidelines

Diagnosis should preferably be based on objective scientific criteria, such as symptom rating scales, electroencephalogram and mechanical devices to assess motor activity.

The child should have a clearly defined condition that is likely to respond to drugs. Few disturbances of wellbeing require treatment, and many behavioural disturbances are due to inappropriate home or school conditions. Sometimes, the motivation for drug use is the convenience of the parents.

All reasonable non-drug interventions, such as social support, special teaching and behaviour modification, should have been proved to be insufficient.

Specialist supervision is nearly always necessary.

Parents must make an informed choice about treatment. Children should be informed or consulted to the level their development allows.

Sedatives, hypnotics and anxiolytics

Sedatives and hypnotics are largely interchangeable descriptive terms, but sedation does not necessarily mean that sleep occurs. Most hypnotics given in divided doses through the day will sedate; similarly, most anxiolytics given in large enough doses will produce sleep.

The duration and type of sleep that people need varies with age, but also markedly between individuals of the same age. Many parents have unrealistic expectations of the sleep their children need. Most sleep disturbances do not require sedatives and much of the demand is generated by parents of normal but wakeful children.

Prescribing sedatives is not a valid alternative to resolving underlying problems by discussion and practical help where possible. In many cases, even where valid indications exist, prescribing sedative drugs does not prove helpful.

Indications for use

The indications for the use of drugs for sleep problems are all controversial.

When a child's sleep problems seriously interfere with normal family life and do not respond to normal parental care and attention, simple behaviour modification involving both parents should be instituted. Occasionally, though not usually, mild sedatives may be useful initially to facilitate the programme. Note that periodic awakening is normal in infants, and drugs should not be used. If one or both parents express feelings of violence, it may be appropriate to admit the child or move the mother, father or family with the child to a controlled situation, such as a hospital room.

Other indications for drug use are severe anxiety states that prove refractory to psychological management; night terrors that are so severe and persistent that they warrant drug therapy; and sedation for medical procedures, such as ophthalmoscopy, and premedication for surgery. Note that routine premedication is not appropriate. Many children respond better to explanation and the presence of parents. Pain due to illness or operative measures requires analgesia, not sedation.

Children with physical illness may require sedatives for brief periods, and children with pruritus due to atopic eczema may be helped at night by sedative prescription.

Prescribing guidelines

Always discuss the possible causes and their resolution by other means, or suggest acceptance of the problem by the parents without therapy.
Give sedatives for short periods only.
Children of most ages require considerably larger than adult weight-related doses.
For young children, the most useful drugs are the short-acting benzodiazepines and alimemazine (trimeprazine). For older children, benzodiazepines are most appropriate.

Alternatives to drugs

As discussed above, drugs should be considered a last-line approach: discussion of the problems and concerns together with the considerable drawbacks of therapy will often help the family, and drugs will not be needed.

Useful drugs

Benzodiazepines

These are effective and extremely safe hypnotics that do not generally interact with other drugs. Side effects are infrequent, but older children tend to have "hangovers" the next morning.
Nitrazepam, diazepam, temazepam and flurazepam are most commonly used. "Hangover" side effects are less common with temazepam than the others, but headache, vertigo, nausea and vomiting occur equally and occasionally with all. The dose should be taken at bedtime.

Oral dose as hypnotics (all ages)

nitrazepam	$250-500 \mu g/kg$ (max. 10 mg)
diazepam	$250-750 \mu g/kg$ (max. 30 mg)
temazepam	$500 \mu g-1 mg/kg$ (max. 30 mg)
flurazepam	$500 \mu g-1 mg/kg$ (max. 30 mg)

Phenothiazines

The most sedating antihistamines are used.
Alimemazine (trimeprazine) is useful for procedural sedation and general hypnosis (particularly if itching disturbs sleep). It is active for

over 12 hours in an oral dose for all ages of 1 mg/kg for daytime sedation (antipruritic) and 3 mg/kg to produce sleep.

It is relatively free of adverse effects, but some children have paradoxical excitement, tremor and insomnia. Anticholinergic effects of dry mouth and blurred vision may occur occasionally. Oculogyric crises occur rarely.

Promethazine is similar to alimemazine (trimeprazine) but perhaps more useful as a daytime sedative and less useful as a hypnotic.

		Oral dose (all ages)
alimemazine (trimeprazine)	daytime sedative bedtime dose	1 mg/kg each day in two doses 3 mg/kg

Note that sudden death has occurred in children under the age of 1 year who were being treated with phenothiazines. They should therefore not be used in this age group.

Anxiolytics

There are very few indications for the use of anxiolytics in children. They should be used only to relieve acute anxiety and related insomnia caused by fear or to prevent anticipatory vomiting with cytotoxic chemotherapy (see section on anti-emetics, p. 38). Other possible use should be directed by a specialist paediatrician/psychiatrist, e.g. behavioural disturbances in the mentally retarded and in acute/chronic anxiety states where their use works as a "holding operation" allowing other forms of psychiatric therapy to be employed.

There is no good evidence that certain drugs are more effective and have fewer adverse effects than others.

	Oral dose as anxiolytics (all ages)
diazepam	100–500 μg/kg each day in three divided doses
lorazepam	50–200 μg/kg each day in three divided doses

Adverse effects can be oversedation and ataxia. Dependence with prolonged use is rare in childhood.

Antidepressants

Indications for use

Endogenous depression is rare in children but more common in adolescents. It should usually be managed by experts. The principal use of antidepressant drugs is therefore in adolescents, occasionally in phobic neurotic states at any age, and more recently as one approach in attention deficit disorder (see section on stimulants, p. 88). For the primary paediatric physician, the only common use of these drugs has been in the management of nocturnal bed-wetting, and tricyclics have been the most commonly used drugs. Their beneficial effects probably relate more to anticholinergic and α-adrenergic than antidepressant properties. However, bed-wetting resolves spontaneously, and there are a number of drawbacks to the use of these drugs (see below). It is arguable whether they should be used for this problem.

Prescribing guidelines

Nocturnal bed-wetting in children under 5 years may be considered to be normal: drug therapy is not indicated.

It is important to attempt to exclude a neurological cause on examination, and urinary tract infection or diabetes mellitus on urine testing.

Overdoses of tricyclics cause cardiac arrhythmias and therapeutic doses may also do so. They must always be dispensed in child-resistant containers. Tablets are preferred to liquids for safety reasons. Note that tricyclic poisoning is responsible for over half the child deaths that result from accidental ingestion, although the source of most of these is adult prescription. These facts should always be considered when prescribing for what is a benign and self-resolving condition.

Drug therapy is less effective than the appropriate use of buzzer alarm devices and should only be tried after other approaches have failed.

Tricyclic antidepressants may not have any effect for up to two or three weeks, although anticholinergic effects are more rapid, as is the benefit in bed-wetting.

Bed-wetting during therapy after initial success (caused by tolerance to the drug) and relapse after drug withdrawal are common.

Alternatives to drugs

Use the reward system: praise and encouragement alone or a coloured star reward system is often effective.

Attention to social factors and family difficulties is important, and appropriate counselling and help may resolve the bed-wetting.

Alarm systems are generally more effective than drugs.

Useful drugs

Tricyclic drugs

All these drugs can be given 2 hours before bedtime. They all have sedative and anticholinergic properties: amitriptyline and imipramine have similar anticholinergic effect; amitriptyline is more sedative than imipramine. There is no evidence that drugs with the greatest anticholinergic effects or with most or least sedative properties are more effective in bed-wetting.

Anticholinergic effects are not usually a problem, but dry mouth, blurred vision, vomiting and constipation can occasionally be bothersome.

Avoid their use in children with cardiac disease (there is a danger of arrhythmias) and epilepsy (the convulsive threshold is lowered). Always prescribe in child-resistant containers.

	Oral dose, 2 h before bedtime	
	5–10 years	*11–16 years*
amitriptyline	10–30 mg	20–60 mg
imipramine	25–50 mg	25–75 mg

All the following adverse effects may occur: sedation, dry mouth, blurred vision, constipation, nausea, fainting, behaviour disturbances and arrhythmias.

Antipsychotics

The treatment of these conditions should usually be initiated by a specialist.

Indications for use

These are:

— schizophrenia and mania
— multiple tics (chorea) and Gilles de la Tourette's syndrome
— developmental disorders
— rarely, emotional and conduct disorders.

Prescribing guidelines

Specialist advice and assessment should always be sought. The lowest possible doses should be used and for short periods only. Adverse effects are severe:

— increase in appetite leads to obesity;
— disorders of movement (dyskinesias) are sometimes serious and, as well as occurring either early or late in treatment, may also occur on withdrawal;
— these drugs may interfere with learning;
— it is not known whether some drugs are safer than others.

Useful drugs

Phenothiazines

These can be used for sedative, anticholinergic or extrapyramidal effects to varying degrees as shown (the ratings of +, ++ and +++ indicate comparative effects and have no absolute values):

	Sedative	Anticholinergic	Extrapyramidal
chlorpromazine, promazine	+++	++	++
periciazine, thioridazine	++	+++	+
fluphenazine, perphenazine, prochlorperazine	+	+	+++

Other drugs

These include butyrophenones (e.g. droperidol, haloperidol), diphenylbutylpiperidines (e.g. pimozide), and thioxanthenes (e.g. chlorprothixene).

Alternatives to drugs

Psychotherapy is less likely to be of help in the conditions for which these drugs are used than in anxiety, depression, insomnia and hyperkinesis.

Stimulants

These should be used only on the recommendation of a specialist paediatrician or child psychiatrist.

Indications for use

Stimulants are for use in children with attention deficit disorder (hyperkinesis). They should not be used in children who are simply described as "active".

Prescribing guidelines

Diagnosis should be based mainly on psychological assessment and parent and teacher reports of severe motor restlessness and inattention, with grossly abnormal results in standardized hyperactivity rating scales.

Obtain a base-line of behaviour before treatment against which to measure changes in behaviour after the treatment is over.

Stimulant drug therapy is complementary to other measures (see below).

Nonspecific spontaneous improvement is fairly common: it may be useful to start medication with a placebo which, if indicated, can be substituted again at a later stage of the active treatment to determine whether it is necessary to continue with specific therapy.

Some drugs (amphetamines and methylphenidate) have a higher black market value than others that are used for this problem, such as tricyclic antidepressants.

Children under 5 years should not be treated with stimulant drugs.

Start with the lowest possible dose: many studies have recommended doses that are too high for some children. Increase the dose gradually, closely monitoring for clinical benefit and adverse effects (reports from parents and teachers are essential). Note that these drugs have long half-lives and accumulate if increment intervals are less than 5–7 days.

Tolerance may develop: "drug holidays" are useful and can be timed to coincide with weekends or vacations.

Alternatives to drugs

These are:

— reassurance and social support
— explanation
— remedial schooling
— specific psychotherapy and behaviour modification.

Useful drugs

Tricyclic antidepressants

Although not specifically stimulants, these are probably the drugs of choice for hyperkinesis in areas where the black market value of methylphenidate and amphetamines is an important consideration. Amitriptyline and imipramine are most commonly used.

	Oral dose
amitriptyline	1–2 mg/kg once daily
imipramine	1–3 mg/kg once daily

Methylphenidate

Because of the frequency and severity of its adverse effects, this drug should not be used by the general practitioner. The adverse effects include anorexia, weight loss, growth inhibition, tearfulness, irritability, insomnia and personality change such as disorientation, aggression and paranoid psychosis. It remains unproven whether catch-up in growth occurs after therapy has stopped.

Drug abuse or dependency with long-term use has not been shown, but the effects have not been evaluated.

Amphetamines

Amphetamines such as dexamphetamine have similar clinical and adverse effects, but have no advantage over methylphenidate. They are not available in some countries. Pyritinol is used in some European countries, but its effectiveness has not been demonstrated.

Anticonvulsants

Seizures in childhood are most commonly either idiopathic or provoked by fever, but the possibility that there may be an underlying disorder must never be neglected. Metabolic problems, such as hypoglycaemia, should always be considered, especially in small babies, and seizures may be a symptom of a wide variety of other diseases. It is also obviously important that breathholding attacks, faints or other "funny turns" should not be mistaken for fits.

By no means all children with seizures require treatment with anticonvulsants and the use of these drugs presents a number of problems. Anticonvulsants are the drugs most commonly implicated in drug interactions in children. They also have many adverse effects, often related closely to drug concentrations in plasma. The wide variability in drug handling in children makes appropriate and risk-free dosing more difficult.

Indications for use

Anticonvulsants should be used to stop an acute seizure. It is desirable to curtail all seizures as soon as possible and especially if they continue for more than one or two minutes and are associated with unconsciousness and possible hypoxia.

Anticonvulsants should also be used for the prophylaxis of recurrent seizures. Treatment is generally considered when there has been more than one clinically significant seizure not provoked by fever or a correctable underlying disorder. This is an important decision as, once started, anticonvulsants usually have to be given for a period of years and effects on the child's development, often subtle, cannot be discounted. Specialist evaluation and investigation is therefore usually indicated before starting treatment.

Prescribing guidelines
Treatment of acute seizures

The approach should be simple, convenient and quickly effective and should, if possible, allow administration by inexperienced personnel including parents. The most useful approaches are shown below.

	Route	Dose	Comment
diazepam	rectal (by rectal tube as liquid, *not* suppository)	5 mg (< 4 years) 10 mg (≧ 4 years)	May be repeated after 10 minutes
	rectal (liquid via syringe)	500 μg/kg all ages (max. 15 mg)	May be repeated after 10 minutes
	intravenous	up to 1 mg/kg (max. 15 mg)	Titrate according to response up to maximum
paraldehyde	deep intramuscular	0.5 ml (< 3 months) 1 ml (3–6 months) 1.5 ml (6–12 months) 2 ml (1–2 years) 3–4 ml (3–5 years) 5–6 ml (6–12 years)	Very painful; rarely, sterile abscesses occur

Control of recurrent seizures

The drugs of most value are carbamazepine, clonazepam, ethosuximide, phenobarbital, phenytoin and sodium valproate (Table 5).

Table 5. Drugs to control recurrent seizures.

Drug	Indications (seizures)	Usual daily dose	No. of divided doses
carbamazepine	Tonic/clonic Simple and complex partial seizures	10–20 mg/kg	2–3
clonazepam	Atonic/akinetic Myoclonic Infantile spasms	50–200 μg/kg	1
ethosuximide	Simple absences	30–50 mg/kg	1
phenobarbital	Tonic/clonic Partial seizures	3–10 mg/kg	1
phenytoin	Tonic/clonic Simple and complex partial seizures	4–9 mg/kg	2
sodium valproate	Tonic/clonic Simple absences Simple and complex partial seizures	20–60 mg/kg	1–3[a]

[a] Although sodium valproate has a short half life (≃ 6–10 h), studies have shown that it has similar efficacy whether taken once or three times daily.

Single drug therapy is effective in over 85% of children and multiple drug therapy is unlikely to be effective in the remainder. A gradual build-up in dose is often necessary. To achieve optimal dosing for children with the minimum of adverse effects, it is often helpful to measure the concentration of the drug in plasma as children vary widely in how they handle these drugs.

If adverse effects or excessive plasma levels occur before acceptable control of convulsions has been achieved, a change to another drug is indicated. The approach involves using each drug to its limits. If A and B are drugs of first choice and C and D are "next best" drugs, start by using A singly and, if unsuccessful, use B singly. C and D should be used singly in turn if convulsions are still not controlled satisfactorily. If control cannot be achieved by one drug alone, it may occasionally be useful to combine drugs, but each combination must be fully assessed in the same way as for single therapy.

Phenobarbital, clonazepam, ethosuximide and probably also sodium valproate can be given in one daily dose and this may improve compliance. Carbamazepine, the benzodiazepines and phenytoin, in low doses, need more frequent administration.

In most cases, therapy may be stopped if 2 or more years have elapsed since the last convulsion. It is advisable to reduce the dose gradually over 2–3 months.

Poor compliance is a major problem in chronic convulsive conditions. Measurement of drug concentrations is helpful in determining whether continuing convulsions are due to this or other causes.

Prevention of febrile convulsions

More than 25% of children who have a convulsion associated with fever go on to have one or more convulsions. Two approaches are used to try to prevent these: measures to reduce fever and the use of anticonvulsants.

Removal of clothing, cooling of the environmental temperature and tepid sponging are all useful in reducing temperature and antipyretic drugs should probably also be used. Paracetamol is preferred in regular doses for about 24–48 hours (see p. 55).

Phenobarbital and sodium valproate have been shown to be partially effective in preventing convulsions when given regularly in maintenance dosage. It is no use introducing them at the time of fever. Diazepam is effective in preventing convulsions when given rectally during febrile episodes.

There is no general agreement as to whether and when prophylactic anticonvulsant therapy should be instituted. Maintenance therapy should probably only be used if two or more of the following factors are present:

— age under 1 year
— underlying neurological disorder
— focal or prolonged seizure (lasting longer than 20 minutes)
— convulsions occurring more often than once every 3–4 months.

Phenobarbital has fewer severe adverse effects than sodium valproate and for this reason may be preferred. On the other hand, the effect on learning and family life of the short attention span and restless, active behaviour that occur in up to 50% of children is an important consideration. Rectal diazepam solution via rectal tube dispensers (see p. 91) introduced during febrile episodes is an alternative approach and obviates the need for regular maintenance therapy. However, it may need to be given more than once during each febrile period and the necessary dose frequency is unknown.

Alternatives to drugs

A ketogenic diet may prove helpful in refractory epilepsy, although the high fat content is unpalatable.

Admission to hospital

There are a number of indications that suggest the child should be admitted to hospital immediately:

— any seizure lasting more than 15 minutes
— any seizure that does not respond to therapy for an acute attack
— seizures that occur in rapid succession
— one or more febrile seizures occurring in children under 2 years of age unless meningitis can be excluded with certainty
— if there is prolonged postictal unconsciousness, confusion or paralysis.

Useful drugs

Carbamazepine

Carbamazepine is effective for the control of tonic/clonic (grand mal) seizures and is the drug of choice for partial seizures of focal origin and of complex type.

It has a short half-life and doses need to be given 2–3 times per day. In infants and toddlers, doses should ideally be given four times per day, but it is hard to space the doses evenly because of their long sleep patterns. A slow-release formulation is available in some countries and allows more convenient frequency of dosing.

Other than when using sustained-release preparations, a compromise reduction in dose frequency often results in wide fluctuations in drug concentrations, with drowsiness and ataxia occurring about 3–5 hours after dosing. These effects are also seen at the beginning of therapy, and it is advisable to build up the dose slowly.

The daily dose should start at 4 mg/kg and increase by 4 mg/kg at three-day intervals so that, by the seventh day, 12 mg/kg is given. Thereafter, increases can be made according to control up to 20 mg/kg. The level at which control is achieved will depend partly on the particular preparation used. The suggested therapeutic concentration range for carbamazepine is 4–12 mg/l (16–50 μmol/l; see p. 23).

In addition to the dose-related adverse effects mentioned above, skin rashes may occur but are less frequent if the dose is increased gradually. They usually resolve after a few days with continued medication but the drug may have to be withdrawn if a rash persists. Carbamazepine has an active metabolite that may be responsible for many of the initial adverse effects. Carbamazepine is an enzyme inducer, and its effect on the metabolism of other drugs given concomitantly must always be considered. It also induces its own metabolism, and the concentration of the parent drug may fall allowing a breakthrough in convulsions during the first weeks of therapy.

Sodium valproate

This drug is effective in most types of epilepsy and in the prophylaxis of febrile convulsions. Because of its adverse effects caution is recommended.

Fatal liver failure has been reported. Haemorrhagic pancreatitis is a rare but important adverse effect. Many children on sodium valproate show a slight rise in serum transaminase values and regular monitoring of liver function seems of no value in predicting acute hepatic necrosis.

The most likely adverse effects are gastrointestinal disturbance (with the liquid, but not the tablets which are enteric-coated), some increase in weight, and thinning or kinking of the hair in about 3–10% of children.

Although the elimination half-life is short ($\simeq$ 6–10 hours) doses may be given once daily as there is no direct relationship between plasma concentration and effect. (Studies have shown that it has a similar effect whether given in one or three doses daily.) For this reason also,

94

monitoring of drug levels is not indicated except to check compliance, and to interpret interactions with other anticonvulsants.

The effective dose varies widely. Most children are controlled in daily doses of between 20 mg/kg and 60 mg/kg given orally for all ages.

Phenobarbital

This is used in the treatment of tonic/clonic and partial seizures, but it is also a first-line drug for febrile convulsion prophylaxis when this is indicated. It is not useful in acute attacks as its penetration of brain tissue is slow.

Its long half-life (over 30–40 hours) allows once-daily dosing, but in chronic use this may result in accumulation which may have adverse effects.

Withdrawal of the drug should be over 2–3 months, as rebound convulsions are more likely to occur with this than with other anticonvulsants.

The elixir is bitter and many infants refuse to swallow it; it contains alcohol, and there is a possibility of disulfiram reactions to other drugs such as latamoxef and metronidazole.

For the longer-term control of convulsions after initial control by other drugs has been achieved, the following dosage is recommended.

	Age	Single dose
Loading dose	< 1 year	15 mg/kg, intramuscular
	1–4 years	15 mg/kg, intramuscular
	5–12 years	12 mg/kg, intramuscular
Repeated dose	1–12 years	3–4 mg/kg each day orally, increasing as necessary up to 10 mg/kg each day

The therapeutic concentration range is 10–35 mg/l (40–140 μmol/l; see p. 23).

Phenobarbital has a sedative effect on some children, but paradoxical hyperkinesis has been described in up to 50% of patients. Short attention span occurs, which is a particularly difficult problem for school and home life. Enzyme induction affects vitamin D metabolism and rickets has been reported in some children.

Phenytoin

Effective in tonic/clonic and partial seizures and in stopping a continuing convulsion. Many feel that chronic use should be avoided as far as possible because of the long-term cosmetic side effects.

95

Begin with an oral dose of 4 mg/kg on the first day, increasing each day by no more than 1 mg/kg up to a daily dose of 9 mg/kg. Dosing once a day is acceptable for some children although for many, and certainly at daily doses of under 6 mg/kg, it is advisable to give two divided doses. Phenytoin should not be administered by the intramuscular route as crystallization occurs and absorption is very slow.

Phenytoin has a narrow therapeutic index, and nystagmus, ataxia and slurred speech may occur as drug metabolism becomes saturated and small increases in dose result in large and disproportionate increases in plasma drug concentrations. Coarsening of the facies, hirsutism and gum hypertrophy are particularly undesirable, and are not clearly related to dose or concentration. Nystagmus, ataxia and slurred speech can be prevented by making small increases in dose and by measuring drug levels in the blood. The therapeutic range of 10–20 mg/l (40–80 μmol/l) is reasonably well established for children (see p. 23).

Primidone

This drug is used in some countries, but does not seem to have important advantages over phenobarbital, which is one of its major metabolites.

Ethosuximide

This is effective for simple absence seizures. If these are complicated by motor seizures and sodium valproate is contraindicated or not effective, combination therapy with another drug will be necessary.

It has a long half-life (over 30 hours) in children of most ages and can be given once daily: 30–50 mg/kg orally for all ages.

Measurement of drug levels in the blood is indicated and useful (the therapeutic range is 40–100 mg/l (280–700 μmol/l); see p. 23).

Gastrointestinal upset and headache are the most frequent adverse effects.

Benzodiazepines

These may be useful in certain types of chronic epilepsy but tolerance[a] develops.

Clonazepam is useful given orally for myoclonic-atonic seizures and given intravenously for status epilepticus. Some children become excessively drowsy and some ataxic. Hypersalivation occurs occasionally.

---

[a] Decreasing effect of a given dose over time.

Oral dosing once a day for chronic conditions is probably appropriate, beginning at 50µg/kg and increasing to 200µg/kg. For acute convulsions, the dose is 50–100µg/kg given intravenously.

Diazepam is a drug of choice for status epilepticus in a rectal or intravenous dose of up to 1 mg/kg according to effect, but the usual effective dose is 150–450µg/kg. Rectal applicators giving a single dose of 5 mg or 10 mg are available and may be used by untrained people such as the parents of epileptic children. Diazepam is less useful in chronic care because tolerance develops.

Both clonazepam and diazepam may cause respiratory depression, but this is rare following rectal administration. This route may therefore be preferred.

Other drugs

Adrenocorticotropic hormone (ACTH) and prednisolone are used in the treatment of infantile spasms. This presentation is an indication that an investigation should be undertaken before starting therapy under specialist control.

Some reports suggest that ACTH is more effective than prednisolone, but this has not been proven. There are drawbacks to its use generally (see pp. 133–134).

	Daily dose
ACTH	20–80 units, intramuscular
tetracosactide	500µg–1 mg, intramuscular
prednisolone	2 mg/kg in 2–3 divided doses, orally

Analgesics

Mild to moderate pain

This will usually respond to the simple analgesics. Paracetamol should be used in preference to acetylsalicylic acid (see p. 56), but in slightly higher doses than those for antipyresis.

Paracetamol

Age	Oral dose	
< 1 year	15 mg/kg	
1–4 years	120–240 mg	no more often than every four hours
5–12 years	250–750 mg	

Acetylsalicylic acid

Age	Oral dose	
1–4 years	75–225 mg	no more often than every four hours
5–12 years	300–450 mg	

The chronic pain of arthritis can be managed with either acetylsalicylic acid or a nonsteroidal anti-inflammatory drug (see later in this section).

Moderate to severe pain

Codeine phosphate

The oral dose, 3 mg/kg each day in four-hourly divided doses, is useful but often causes constipation in repeated dosing.

Dihydrocodeine tartrate

This is more potent than codeine phosphate but similarly constipating. The oral dose is 500 μg–1 mg/kg every 4–6 hours as needed.

Severe pain

Narcotic analgesics will usually be required, and these should be used only under close supervision. All carry serious risks of respiratory depression, and this is a greater problem in acute use.

Tolerance and dependence[a] occur, but these are not a big problem in the circumstances in which these drugs are used repeatedly: terminal care. In chronic pain, it is important to give analgesics regularly *before* pain develops; much smaller doses are then effective. To maintain effective analgesia, the dose and frequency have to be increased gradually as tolerance develops.

All cause constipation and laxatives are usually required.

The choice of drug is a matter of the personal preference of the user: morphine is widely used.

Severe bone pain may be helped by the addition of nonsteroidal anti-inflammatory drugs (see p. 155).

Morphine

This often causes nausea and vomiting, which can be reduced by giving a phenothiazine, such as chlorpromazine, concurrently. Euphoria and "mental detachment" occur but they may be regarded as beneficial effects.

The morphine dose may be given orally, subcutaneously, intramuscularly or intravenously. Start with a dose of $200 \mu g/kg$ (for all ages), every 4 hours initially, thereafter titrating dose and frequency to effect. The oral route is preferred for repeated dosing. Chlorpromazine ($500 \mu g$–1 mg/kg) will usually prevent vomiting when given every 6–8 hours.

Methadone

This may be given orally, subcutaneously, intramuscularly or intravenously. Start with a dose of $100 \mu g/kg$ (for all ages) and titrate as for morphine.

Pethidine

This is useful for acute severe pain, particularly for renal or biliary colic, but is not recommended for chronic use because of the accumulation of toxic metabolites. The daily dose is $500 \mu g$–1.5 mg/kg.

Carbamazepine

This may be useful for neuralgic pain.

---

[a] Physical need for a drug following its withdrawal.

Drugs for the treatment of migraine

Migraine occurs most often in the later years of childhood, but is also seen in young children. The cardinal symptom is recurrent paroxysmal headache with periods of freedom and at least two of the following:

— unilateral site
— nausea or vomiting
— visual aura
— family history of migraine

Migraine in childhood often takes atypical forms, however, such as recurrent vomiting or abdominal pain without headache. Diagnosis is then difficult. The treatment of an acute attack and the measures used in prophylaxis are best considered separately.

Treatment of Acute Attack

Most children prefer to lie down in a quiet, dark room.

Analgesia

Treatment should be started as soon as possible. Paracetamol is the drug of choice and should be given in the doses indicated for mild to moderate pain (see p. 98). The effervescent preparations may be more acceptable and better absorbed as gastric stasis is usually present.

Note that ergotamine tartrate and its derivatives are probably best avoided in childhood because of their troublesome and sometimes dangerous adverse effects, such as ergotism and confusion.

Caffeine is often used in combination products for the treatment of migraine.

Anti-emesis

Metoclopramide is the the drug of choice as it increases the gastric emptying rate and so improves analgesic absorption. The oral route may be effective if given before vomiting has started. If vomiting has started, the intramuscular or intravenous route should be used and is often required. Combination preparations with paracetamol may be useful and convenient for older children, although the variation of one drug dose relative to that of the other drug is not possible. Children are more prone to dystonic reactions than adults (for treatment, see section on antihistamines, p. 151).

Age	Dose (oral, intramuscular or intravenous)
<1 year	1 mg twice daily (not for migraine)
1–2 years	1 mg three times daily
3–4 years	2 mg twice or three times daily
5–12 years	2–5 mg three times daily

Metoclopramide also comes in the form of tablets or sachets with paracetamol: metoclopramide 5 mg/paracetamol 500 mg.

Prophylaxis

Alternatives to drugs

These approaches should always be tried first and used alongside drug therapy if it is indicated:

— reassurance and reduction of avoidable stress;

— avoidance of factors known to trigger attacks in an individual patient, such as specific foods (oranges, chocolate, cheese, yoghurt), colouring agents, preservatives, perfumes, sunlight, excessive exertion or delayed or missed meals.

Indications for drug use

Indications are difficult to define because the condition is benign and intermittent, and continuous drug therapy is inconvenient and may have adverse effects that outweigh potential benefits.

It is reasonable to give therapy:

— for a child who has more than two serious attacks a month;

— when the attacks are not adequately alleviated by the above measures.

Therapy for two or three months may be all that is required in the first instance.

Useful drugs

Pizotifen

This is an antiserotoninergic and antihistaminic agent which may be slightly more effective than beta-blockers and is probably the drug of choice. The daily dose for 5–12-year-olds is $500\mu g$–1.5 mg in one or two divided doses.

β-adrenergic blocking agents

Propranolol is effective in about 60% of adults, although the response rate may not be similar in children. Some but not all other beta-blockers are effective. Because of the variation in the extent of first-pass metabolism in different patients, dosage guidelines are imprecise. The suggested oral dose in 5–12-year-olds is 1–4 mg/kg each day in divided doses.

Analgesics

Paracetamol may be effective if given regularly, in two thirds of the dose used in the treatment of mild to moderate pain (see p. 98), three times daily for all ages.

α-adrenergic agonists

Clonidine seems less effective in children than in adults. Methysergide has adverse effects, notably retroperitoneal fibrosis, which suggest it should not be used.

Infections and infestations

Antibacterial agents and their use

Indications for use

Laboratory diagnoses are seldom available when therapy commences, and so antibacterial therapy should be chosen on the basis of the organisms most commonly involved. Cover of uncommon pathogens is necessary only for life-threatening infections, particularly in hospital.

Prescribing guidelines

Oral therapy is adequate, except for potentially life-threatening infection. It is cheap and easy to organize. The parenteral route is indicated if there is vomiting or severe diarrhoea.

Compared with many other drugs used in children, most of these agents have wide therapeutic indices enabling doses to be given in a less specific and non-weight-related manner.

Data sheets recommend that some agents be given four times daily. There is no evidence that administration three times daily is inferior in minor or moderate infection, and except for life-threatening infection this approach is appropriate.

The duration of drug therapy depends on the nature of the infection and the response to treatment. Many liquids are dispensed in containers that will allow 20 doses, and 7 days' therapy is therefore more practical than the 10 days sometimes recommended. Evidence is increasing that shorter than usual courses are just as effective for certain infections.

Adverse effects

Antibiotics may select out resistant strains in the bowel flora and also encourage oral thrush, which is less likely with narrow spectrum agents.

Diarrhoea is common, but severe staphylococcal enteritis or pseudomembranous enterocolitis caused by *Clostridium difficile* are rare. Both of these conditions give rise to other signs and symptoms.

Rashes due to hypersensitivity often occur. If they do, withdraw the drug, unless the infection is life-threatening.

103

Useful drugs

Penicillins

Penicillin G, its prolonged action derivatives, phenoxymethylpenicillin and pheneticillin are active against most *Streptococcus* spp. (including *S. pneumoniae*) and *Clostridium* spp., but only some *Staphylococcus* and *Neisseria* spp.

Ampicillin and its esters and amoxicillin are, in addition, active against *S. faecalis*, most *Escherichia coli* strains, some *Klebsiella* and *Proteus* spp., and about 90% of *Haemophilus influenzae* strains (this figure varies according to local resistance patterns).

A combination of clavulanic acid (a β-lactamase inhibitor) and amoxicillin (not available in all countries) is more active than amoxicillin alone against urinary infections caused by gram-negative bacteria and other resistant organisms, including *H. influenzae*.

Flucloxacillin, cloxacillin and dicloxacillin are antistaphylococcal drugs with some activity against *Streptococcus* spp., including *S. pneumoniae* but excluding *S. faecalis*.

There are only occasional indications for continued therapy with the other injectable penicillins that are used in hospital.

The adverse effects of the penicillins include rashes and hypersensitive reactions (including anaphylaxis; see p. 103) with cross-allergy between the penicillins. However, rashes due to the ampicillin group are not always due to penicillin allergy, e.g. the rash of infectious mononucleosis. Avoid the esters of ampicillin in chronic renal insufficiency to prevent the toxic effects of raised blood levels of ester moiety.

Cephalosporins

Cefalexin, cefradine, cefaclor and cefadroxil should be given orally. These have the same antibacterial spectrum as ampicillin (though they are not active against *S. faecalis*) but, in addition, they are active against *Staphylococcus* spp. and many other gram-negative bacteria. Cefaclor is also active against *H. influenzae*. Some 10% of patients who are allergic to penicillin are also sensitive to cephalosporins.

Tetracycline

Tetracycline is useful in *Brucella* and *Rickettsia* infections. It may also be used topically on skin, eyes and external auditory meatus. It may be used orally to treat acne in the older child.

It is contraindicated in young children (under 8 years) because it causes staining of teeth, enamel hypoplasia and inhibition of bone growth. Alternative agents suitable for systemic action are available for all common infections.

Erythromycin

This has similar activity to phenoxymethylpenicillin and pheneticillin but it also works against *Bordetella pertussis, Campylobacter jejuni, Mycoplasma pneumoniae, Chlamydia trachomatis* and *Legionella pneumophila.*

The estolate produces higher levels of erythromycin than other salts with similar weight-related doses — its kinetic profile is such that it allows dosing every 12 hours.

Avoid giving treatment for more than 14 days with estolate (cholestatic jaundice has been reported with prolonged therapy).

Lincomycin and clindamycin

These are active against *Staphylococcus* spp., most *Streptococcus* spp. and anaerobic bacteria. They should be used mainly for bone and joint infections and are best confined to hospital use. They occasionally precipitate pseudomembranous colitis and should therefore be avoided in infections other than those mentioned above.

Chloramphenicol

This is active against gram-positive and gram-negative organisms, notably *Haemophilus influenzae.* Its adverse effects limit its blind use to life-threatening infection, particularly meningitis, typhoid fever or epiglottitis. These effects are dose-related (concentration-related) reversible marrow suppression and idiosyncratic or non-dose-related irreversible aplasia. Grey syndrome (circulatory collapse and respiratory depression) is concentration-related and occurs mainly in the newborn but may occur in older children.

Aminoglycosides

These have a broad spectrum of activity, some including *Pseudomonas* spp. They are not absorbed orally and most are indicated only in hospital.

Streptomycin is active against *Mycobacterium tuberculosis.* Topical neomycin and framycetin are used for eye and skin infections and for otitis externa. Avoid the topical use of gentamicin to prevent resistance from emerging, which would decrease its usefulness systemically.

The adverse effects of aminoglycosides include concentration-related ototoxicity and nephrotoxicity, which may occur even with inhalation therapy in cystic fibrosis. Serum concentrations must be monitored.

Note that topical ear preparations should not be used when the eardrum is perforated.

There is a risk of hypersensitivity, particularly with topical neomycin and framycetin.

Fusidic acid

This is a narrow-spectrum antistaphylococcal agent used for bone and joint infections.

Sulfonamides

Their activity against urinary pathogens, *Neisseria meningitidis* and other pathogens is now significantly reduced by resistant strains, and because of this there are few indications for "blind" uses of these drugs. Sulfadiazine may be applied topically to burns. Topical preparations are also useful for some eye infections. Rashes may occur, but erythema multiforme is rare.

Trimethoprim

It is used alone for urinary tract infections or in combination with sulfamethoxazole (as co-trimoxazole) for minor respiratory infections, urinary infections and invasive salmonellosis. The combination has little advantage over trimethoprim alone for the treatment of urinary tract infections. Resistance to sulfonamide, and the incidence of adverse effects due to the sulfonamide component suggests single trimethoprim therapy is most appropriate.

Metronidazole

This antiprotozoal agent is active against anaerobic bacteria, such as those implicated in gingivitis, infections after bowel surgery and perianal abscess. It is widely used in hospital for prophylaxis in bowel surgery.

Nitrofurantoin

This urinary antiseptic causes gastrointestinal upset. It is contraindicated in renal impairment.

Rifampicin

This antituberculous drug acts against *Neisseria meningitidis*. It is used for prophylaxis and the eradication of the carrier state in meningococcal and *Haemophilus* infections, and as the first-line treatment of tuberculosis in combination with other agents. It colours saliva, tears and urine brick red, causes gastrointestinal upset and can alter liver function and cause jaundice.

Isoniazid

This is a first-line drug against tuberculosis. The adverse effect of peripheral neuritis (preventable by pyridoxine) has not been reported in children but it has occurred in adults. Gastrointestinal upset, occasionally hepatotoxic, and rarely psychoses are other problems.

Ethambutol

This can be used in the initial stage of antituberculous therapy, pending the results of tests of the patient's sensitivity to it. It may cause optic neuritis, so advise the patient to report visual disturbances and arrange ophthalmic examinations on commencement and thereafter three-monthly in the rare instances that this agent is continued.

Pyrazinamide

This penetrates the meninges well and is therefore particularly useful in tuberculous meningitis. Its adverse effects are hepatotoxicity and urticaria.

Prophylaxis

The aim of antibiotic prophylaxis is to prevent a specific infection in an individual who is at risk.

Meningococcal infections

Household contacts of patients with meningococcal infection often have a colonized nasopharynx and some contacts develop serious infections. It is also possible that organisms may linger in contacts and reinfect the original patient following recovery.

Colonization can be prevented by eradicating the organism with antibiotics in a concentration in nasopharyngeal secretions sufficient to kill the organisms.

Treat the entire household regardless of age with rifampicin, sulfadimidine or sulfadiazine. Use sulfadimidine or sulfadiazine only when there is evidence that the isolate is sensitive to these drugs.

	Age	Eradication dose	
rifampicin	< 1 year	15 mg/kg	
	1–4 years	15 mg/kg	in two divided doses
	5–12 years	15 mg/kg	each day for 2 days
	> 12 years	1.2 g	

	Age	
sulfadimidine	< 1 year	125 mg
	1–4 years	250 mg
	5–12 years	500 mg	twice daily for 5 days
	> 12 years	1 g

sulfadiazine	1–4 years	500 mg once daily for 2 days
	5–12 years	500 mg twice daily for 2 days
	> 12 years	1 g twice daily for 2 days

Note that rifampicin induces hepatic metabolizing enzymes and increases the metabolism of oral contraceptive hormones. This could lead to pregnancy when given in prolonged dosage for tuberculosis. Whether this risk is present with two-day eradication therapy is not known.

Haemophilus influenzae infections

In severe infections and when children under 5 years of age are in contact, treat all the family members with rifampicin, as in the case of meningococcal infection (see above), but for 4 days.

Rheumatic fever

Patients who have had carditis are at risk of a further attack when infected with *Streptococcus pyogenes*. Prophylaxis with phenoxymethylpenicillin should continue at least until the patient reaches 21 years of age (and perhaps for life).

	Age	Prophylactic dose	
phenoxymethylpenicillin	1–4 years	125 mg	
	5–12 years	250 mg	once daily
	> 12 years	500 mg	

In patients allergic to penicillin, use erythromycin (as stearate).

	Age	Prophylactic dose	
erythromycin (stearate)	1–4 years	125 mg	
	5–12 years	250 mg	twice daily
	>12 years	500 mg	

When compliance is poor use benzathine benzylpenicillin.

	Age	Prophylactic dose	
benzathine benzylpenicillin	<5 years	229 mg	
	5–12 years	458 mg	every 4 weeks
	>12 years	916 mg	

Note that resistant strains of *Streptococcus viridans* develop in the oral flora within a few days of starting therapy (see prophylaxis against endocarditis below).

Endocarditis

Patients with congenital valve lesions, septal defects, ductus arteriosus and rheumatic valve damage are prone to endocarditis, which may follow dental treatment or operations on other "dirty" areas.

Prophylaxis should produce serum concentrations greatly in excess of those necessary to kill the organisms that enter the blood stream. Concentrations should peak at the time of bacteraemia (arising from, for example, scaling of teeth or tooth extraction).

A prophylactic dose of amoxicillin should be given to those who have not received penicillin in the previous 4 weeks. Large dose sachets are available.

	Age	First oral dose (1 h before procedure)	Second oral dose (6 h later)
amoxicillin	<10 years	1.5 g	750 mg
	>10 years	3 g	1.5 g

For allergic individuals and those who have been treated with phenoxymethylpenicillin in the last 4 weeks, use erythromycin (as stearate).

	Age	First dose (1 h before procedure)	Second dose (6 h later)
erythromycin (stearate)	<10 years	750 mg	250 mg
	>10 years	1.5 g	500 mg

Infections due to Streptococcus pneumoniae

Patients who have sickle cell disease or have had a splenectomy are prone to pneumococcal pneumonia, and septicaemia and meningitis due to *Streptococcus pneumoniae*. Patients who present or relapse with nephrotic syndrome, particularly those with ascites, are prone to peritonitis due to *S. pneumoniae*. The incidence of these infections can be reduced by prophylaxis with phenoxymethylpenicillin (or erythromycin, if patients are allergic to penicillin, or benzathine benzylpenicillin if compliance is poor). The prophylactic dose is as for rheumatic fever (see pp. 108–109).

As compliance with regular therapy is often poor, pneumococcal vaccine should be used in addition in children aged 2 years and over. However, the vaccine contains only the pneumococcal serotypes responsible for 80% of serious infection.

Treatment

Sore throat

Most cases of sore throat are viral and do not require antibiotics, but it is not possible clinically to differentiate viral from bacterial infection. There is a greater chance that infection is streptococcal if there is a high fever, marked inflammation with exudate or tender cervical glands. Antibiotic therapy hastens resolution slightly in streptococcal cases and reduces infectivity, but the organism is not always eradicated.

In most cases, no drug therapy is indicated. In the few cases in which there is a high suspicion of streptococcal origin, it is reasonable to give phenoxymethylpenicillin or erythromycin (erythromycin is the drug of choice where the patient is hypersensitive to penicillin).

	Age	*Oral dose*	
phenoxymethylpenicillin	< 1 year	62.5 mg	three times daily for 10 days before meals
	1–5 years	125 mg	
	6–12 years	250 mg	
erythromycin (stearate)	< 1 year	62.5 mg	three times daily for 10 days
	1–5 years	125 mg	
	6–12 years	250 mg	

Failure to eradicate *Streptococcus pyogenes*, with resulting recurrent attacks of tonsillitis, may be due to the destruction of penicillin-type antibiotics by β-lactamase enzymes produced by the normal bacterial flora of the mouth. In such cases give amoxicillin/clavulanic acid, or a cephalosporin. The amoxicillin/clavulanic acid ratio for younger children (4 : 1) is different from that for older children (2 : 1).

	Age	Dose	
amoxicillin/ clavulanic acid	3–12 months	31 mg/7.6 mg	
	1–2 years	62.5 mg/15.5 mg	three times daily for 10–14 days
	2–4 years	125 mg/31 mg	
	5–12 years	250 mg/125 mg	

Otitis media

The commonest causes of otitis media are *Haemophilus influenzae* and *Streptococcus pneumoniae* in the under-fives and *S. pneumoniae* in the over-fives. *S. pyogenes*, *Staphylococcus* spp. and other bacteria are less common.

Pain is usually present when antibiotic therapy is indicated: when the drum is generally red, dull with loss of light reflex or bulging. Other conditions of the drum, such as partial redness or vessel injection, need not be treated with antibiotics.

Decongestants are widely used but not of proven value. Treatment, where indicated, should include both analgesics (paracetamol; see p. 55) and antibiotics (amoxicillin or co-trimoxazole).

	Age	Oral dose	
amoxicillin	< 1 year	62.5 mg	
	1–4 years	125 mg	three times daily for 7 days
	5–12 years	250 mg	

	Age	Oral dose (trimethoprim/sulfamethoxazole)	
co-trimoxazole	< 1 year	20 mg/100 mg	
	1–4 years	40 mg/200 mg	twice daily for 7 days
	5–12 years	80 mg/400 mg	

Note that phenoxymethylpenicillin has a lower success rate in children under 5 years and erythromycin is less effective in all age groups than either amoxicillin or co-trimoxazole. Check tympanic membranes after treatment. Failed resolution is usually due to resistant *H. influenzae*. Give amoxicillin plus clavulanic acid or cefaclor for 10–14 days (for doses, see above and p. 113).

111

Croup and epiglottitis

In most cases, inspiratory stridor is due to viral laryngotracheobronchitis. It is rarely due to epiglottitis, but this must always be considered. Epiglottitis is a potentially life-threatening infection in children, particularly those under 4 years old, and is due to *H. influenzae*. It is differentiated clinically from other infective causes of respiratory stridor by:

— rapid onset, usually a few hours

— drooling (open-mouthed, worried look is characteristic)

— high fever

— toxic appearance of child (there is usually associated septicaemia)

— "muffled" voice, since there is no laryngitis.

The management of likely epiglottitis involves transport to hospital immediately. Stay with the child during the journey. Do not attempt to visualize the larynx as complete obstruction may be precipitated. Be prepared to do an emergency tracheostomy if the child's airway does become completely obstructed.

Pertussis

The causative agent, *Bordetella pertussis*, causes necrosis of the bronchial epithelium and mucus accumulation before the classic paroxysms of coughing become manifest. Antibiotics do not modify the protracted course of the disease and are of use to the affected individual only when there is a concomitant pneumonia. Certain antibiotics penetrate the respiratory tract, eradicate the carrier state and reduce infectivity.

The agent of choice is erythromycin.

	Age	Oral dose	
erythromycin	< 1 year	62.5 mg	
	1–4 years	125 mg	} three times daily for 10 days
	5–12 years	250 mg	

Co-trimoxazole is an alternative eradicating drug, but amoxicillin is unreliable.

The place of cough suppressants is controversial but the opiate analogues may be helpful and phenobarbital and salbutamol have advocates.

Pneumonia

Bacterial pneumonia may be primary or follow a virus infection. *Streptococcus pneumoniae* is the commonest cause, but *Haemophilus influenzae* is important, especially in the under-fives and those children with chronic chest disorders such as cystic fibrosis.

Pneumonia due to *Staphylococcus aureus* is much less common but more severe and dangerous, especially in those under 2 years old. It may be a complication of measles and influenza and therapy given for bacterial pneumonia following these virus infections should include an antistaphylococcal agent.

Pneumonia due to *Mycoplasma pneumoniae* responds to erythromycin.

Most mild cases of pneumonia can be managed at home. For children under 5 years old use amoxicillin and for those over 5 years old use phenoxymethylpenicillin, pheneticillin or erythromycin.

In severe cases, children of all ages should be given amoxicillin and flucloxacillin or cloxacillin, unless there is an epidemic of pneumonia due to *M. pneumoniae*, when erythromycin should be used.

If cystic fibrosis or staphylococci are suspected, combine the following doses of amoxicillin with equal doses of cloxacillin and/or flucloxacillin, or use cefaclor alone.

	Age	Dose	
amoxicillin, cloxacillin or flucloxacillin	< 1 year	62.5 mg	three times daily
	1–4 years	125 mg	
	5–12 years	250 mg	
cefaclor	< 1 year	62.5 mg	three times daily
	1–4 years	125 mg	
	5–12 years	250 mg	

Seven days' therapy is usually sufficient, except in those children with cystic fibrosis or bronchiectasis.

Urinary tract infection

Urinary tract infection is common in childhood; it may be asymptomatic, produce a nonspecific illness or have obvious urinary symptoms and signs. It must be suspected whenever unexplained infection is present. It is important that the diagnosis be confirmed in the laboratory. All children who have had a proven urinary infection should be referred for exclusion of structural abnormality or reflux nephropathy.

Treat with trimethoprim, amoxicillin or oral cephalosporin for 7 days or for 3 days after the urine is clear of organisms. Shorter courses may also be effective.

	Age	Dose	
trimethoprim	< 1 year	25 mg	⎫
	1–4 years	50 mg	⎬ twice daily
	5–12 years	100 mg	⎭

amoxicillin	< 1 year	62.5 mg	⎫
	1–4 years	125 mg	⎬ three times daily
	5–12 years	250 mg	⎭

oral cephalosporin	< 1 year	62.5 mg	⎫
	1–4 years	125 mg	⎬ three times daily
	5–12 years	250 mg	⎭

Prophylaxis may be recommended after investigation if the child has repeated infections or if a structural abnormality is present. The need for prophylaxis should be reviewed annually.

To prevent reinfection the agent chosen is normally given at night (so that it is retained in the bladder) at a quarter of the total daily dose recommended for the treatment of established infection. Trimethoprim is the drug of first choice.

Tuberculosis

Specialist investigation is indicated, including skin testing (except after BCG when interpretation is difficult) and radiological investigation.

In the initial phase of therapy, the aims are to kill the mycobacteria rapidly and to use a combination of agents that will minimize the problems of antibiotic resistance. Rifampicin and isoniazid are often supplemented by ethambutol (or pyrazinamide in extrapulmonary infections, especially tuberculous meningitis) during this phase, which lasts for 8–12 weeks.

Continued therapy with isoniazid and rifampicin for a further 7 months is usually satisfactory, once the sensitivity pattern is known.

	Dose	
isoniazid	10–15 mg/kg (max. 300 mg)	⎫
rifampicin	15 mg/kg (max. 400 mg)	⎬ once daily
ethambutol	15 mg/kg	⎬
pyrazinamide	20–30 mg/kg	⎭

For their adverse effects, see p. 106–107.

114

It is essential that compliance with therapy is regularly checked. This should include demonstrations by the parent of the number of tablets taken and home visits to check that stocks of drugs are compatible with compliance. Warn the parents that on rifampicin therapy the urine will be red.

Children who are found to have a positive skin test, but no clinical or radiological evidence of infection, should be given antituberculous therapy. Unless the organism is insensitive, isoniazid alone for 6 months is satisfactory.

Suspected tuberculous meningitis or miliary tuberculosis is an indication for urgent hospital admission.

Antifungal drugs

Flucytosine

This is recommended for use in systemic infections only.

Griseofulvin

This is active against dermatophytic fungi of the genera *Trichophyton*, *Microsporum* and *Epidermophyton*. It is inactive topically but is well absorbed from the gastrointestinal tract. It incorporates into keratin and prevents the infection of new hair, nails and skin. Prolonged treatment is therefore required. The dose is 10 mg/kg each day in two divided doses for all ages, preferably administered with meals (microcrystalline griseofulvin). Its adverse effects are uncommon but include nausea, rashes and photosensitivity.

Amphotericin B

This is active against *Candida albicans*, and other yeasts and fungi. It should be used topically for infections of the skin and mucous membranes. It is not absorbed from the gastrointestinal tract. It may also be administered parenterally but this route is not discussed here.

Form	Dose (topical use, all ages)
suspension (100 mg/ml)	100–200 mg left in the mouth after feeds, at least four times daily
lozenges (10 mg)	10 mg after feeds 4–8 times daily
tablets (100 mg)	suspension and lozenges recommended instead
lotion (30 mg/ml)	2–3 applications daily
ointment and cream (30 mg/g)	2–3 applications daily

Nystatin

This is active when used topically on skin and mucous membranes against *Candida albicans* and other yeasts. It is not absorbed from the gastrointestinal tract.

Form	Dose (all ages)
suspension (100 000 units/ml)	200 000–500 000 units after feeds or a mouthwash at least four times daily
tablets (500 000 units)	500 000 units at least four times daily
ointment (100 000 units/g)	2–3 applications daily

Miconazole

This is active against dermatophytic fungi and yeasts. Use topically only, e.g. for oral thrush. The gel formulation is more easily applied than the suspension.

The dose for oral gel (25 mg/ml) is 50 mg after food and mouthwashing for all ages; use at least four times daily.

Ketoconazole

This has the same activity as miconazole. Note that because of reports of hepatotoxicity and death, its use should be reserved for serious systemic infections only. Its adverse effects are nausea, pruritus and hepatitis. Discontinue therapy immediately if hepatitis develops.

Clotrimazole

This is a broad-spectrum antifungal agent, effective against tinea pedis and other tinea infections, when used topically. Cream 1%, solution 1% (for hairy areas), spray 1% (for hairy areas), or powder 1% should be applied 2–3 times daily for all ages. Its adverse effects are pruritus and skin sensitivity.

Antiviral drugs

Indications for use

Most virus infections are not effectively treated by the drugs available at present, but there are a small number of infections for which therapy is probably effective and indicated. They are:

— herpesviral encephalitis;
— severe herpes stomatitis and herpes stomatitis that is spreading and with underlying atopic eczema;
— zoster in immunosuppressed states, e.g. in children receiving cytotoxic therapy;
— herpesviral or zoster ocular disease; and
— genital herpes.

Prophylaxis may also be given against herpetic infections in immunocompromised children.

Useful drugs

Aciclovir

It is active against human (alpha) herpesvirus 1, 2 and 3. Its action depends on a viral enzyme converting aciclovir to a compound that has a specific virucidal effect. This selective action (on virus infected cells only) is responsible for its low toxicity.

Age	Oral dose	
<2 years	100 mg	five times daily at four-hourly intervals
>2 years	200 mg	

Ophthalmic ointment 3% should be applied five times daily.

Idoxuridine

It is active against herpesviral vesicular dermatitis and zoster, but resistant isolates occur. It is less effective than aciclovir or vidarabine. It can be used topically for herpesviral ocular disease; it is too toxic for systemic use.

Vidarabine

It has similar activity to aciclovir but it is not absorbed from the gastrointestinal tract. It is used to treat herpesviral keratoconjunctivitis. Ointment 3% should be applied five times daily and eye ointment 0.5% every 4 hours.

Drugs for intestinal parasites

Giardiasis

Giardia lamblia is a protozoan with worldwide distribution, which should be treated with metronidazole.

	Age	Dose	
metronidazole	< 1 year	200–400 mg	
	1–4 years	600 mg	once daily for 3 days
	5–12 years	1.2 g	

If this therapy fails to stop the symptoms or there is nausea, reduce the dose by half and continue the treatment for 10 days. If the therapy fails, use tinidazole.

	Age	Single dose
tinidazole	< 1 year	500 mg
	1–4 years	750 mg
	5–12 years	1–1.5 g

The adverse effects of both drugs are nausea, drowsiness, headache, rashes and darkening of urine.

Threadworms

Enterobius vermicularis lays eggs in the perianal region at night causing pruritus ani. Scratching contaminates the hands and sucking the fingers perpetuates the cycle. Break this cycle with sound personal hygiene: showering/bathing in the morning; washing the hands thoroughly and scrubbing under the nails after using the toilet and before meals; clothes should be washed at high temperature. All members of the family require treatment.

A single 100-mg dose of mebendazole for all ages is the most convenient effective therapy, but mebendazole is not licensed for children under 2 years. Alternatively, piperazine may be used. It is available as the following salts: piperazine hydrate (100 mg), piperazine citrate (125 mg) and piperazine phosphate (104 mg).

	Age	Dose	
piperazine hydrate	< 1 year	250–500 mg	
	1–4 years	750 mg	once daily for 7 days
	5–12 years	1.5 g	

Note that piperazine citrate elixir is highly concentrated (750 mg/5 ml) and is therefore sometimes given to children in an excessive dose, causing a characteristic dramatic and worrying ataxia, "worm wobble". It should not be used in children with epilepsy and in those who have had febrile convulsions.

Roundworms

Infestation with *Ascaris lumbricoides* is less common than with threadworm, but both are sensitive to the same agents. Mebendazole should be given orally: 100 mg twice daily for 3 days for all ages over 2 years old. Note that the dosage is different to that for threadworm therapy.

Piperazine hydrate may also be given.

	Age	Oral dose	
piperazine hydrate	< 1 year	1 g	
	1–4 years	2 g	once
	5–12 years	3 g	

Bephenium is a second-line drug.

Hookworm (*Necator* spp. and *Ancylostoma* spp.)

Hookworms reside in the small intestine and cause iron deficiency anaemia. Treatment is required both to kill the parasite and to counteract the anaemia. Like many other worms, they are more often found in immigrants, and infection with multiple parasites is common. Laboratory confirmation and identification is required before starting therapy.

Mebendazole should be given orally: 100 mg twice a day for 3 days for all ages over 2 years.

Other worms and parasites

Laboratory confirmation and identification are required. *Trichuris trichuria* may be treated with mebendazole as for roundworms.

Tiabendazole may be given to treat the following conditions:

	Length of treatment	Oral dose (twice daily)		
		< 1 year	1–4 years	5–12 years
dracunculiasis	1 day			
strongyloidiasis	2 days			
cutaneous larva migrans	2 days	250–500 mg	750 mg	1 g
trichinosis	2–4 days			
visceral larva migrans (*Toxocara* spp.)	7 days			

Tapeworm

Beef tapeworm (*Taenia saginata*) and pork tapeworm (*T. solium*) should be treated with niclosamide.

	Age	Oral dose	
niclosamide	1–4 years	500 mg	
	5–10 years	1 g	once
	> 10 years	1.5 g	

Drugs for malaria

Malaria should be suspected if fever develops after return from an area with malaria, even if adequate prophylaxis has been maintained. Children who may be suffering from malaria should be referred to a specialist immediately.

Prophylaxis

Prophylaxis should be considered for all children travelling to malaria-endemic areas. Information about the risk of malaria and the presence of resistant strains should be obtained from a specialist. Resistant strains of *Plasmodium falciparum* are constantly changing; resistance to chloroquine is widespread and also occurs to most other agents in the Far East, Central and South America, East Africa and occasionally in other parts of Africa.

Where resistance occurs, a pyrimethamine and dapsone combination should be given. If *P. vivax* is also present, chloroquine should be given in addition. Proguanil is safe to give in glucose-6-phosphate dehydrogenase deficiency, but there may be localized resistance of *P. falciparum* to the drug in areas where it is not resistant to chloroquine.

Prophylaxis should start 1 week before departure, continue throughout the stay and must not be stopped until at least 4 weeks after return. For routine prophylaxis give chloroquine or proguanil.

	Age	*Dose*
chloroquine	>1 year	5 mg/kg once weekly

proguanil	<1 year	25–50 mg	
	1–5 years	50–100 mg	once daily
	6–12 years	100–150 mg	

For resistant *P. falciparum* use a pyrimethamine and dapsone combination.

	Age	Weekly dose
pyrimethamine/dapsone	< 1 year	suitable formulation not available
(12.5 mg) (100 mg)	1–5 years	6.25 mg/50 mg
	6–12 years	9.975 mg/75 mg

If there is a risk of *P. vivax* infection, give chloroquine in addition to pyrimethamine/dapsone.

The adverse effects of chloroquine are nausea, vomiting, rashes and pruritus. It may cause corneal and retinal changes after prolonged high doses, and these may be irreversible. Proguanil may cause mild gastro-intestinal intolerance, and pyrimethamine may cause haemopoiesis suppression with prolonged treatment.

The endocrine system

Insulin

Background to therapeutic approach

A child with suspected diabetes mellitus, even if not ketotic, should be referred to hospital immediately.

Diabetes in childhood is almost always insulin-dependent: oral hypoglycaemic agents have no place in the management of Type 1 diabetes. Insulin has been available since 1922. Traditionally beef and pork insulins, which have similar potency, were used in mixed preparations. Both are antigenic in man, though pork less so than beef because it varies from the human insulin molecule by only one amino acid whereas beef varies by three.

Highly purified preparations greatly reduce this antigenicity and abolish some local complications such as lipoatrophy. Although there is as yet no proven long-term benefit, all children should be treated with highly purified preparations in view of the long duration of treatment that can be anticipated.

Human insulin has recently become available, made either by the chemical modification of pork insulin or by biosynthesis. There is to date no evidence that human insulin is superior to the highly purified pork or beef preparations, but it is still less antigenic and it seems wise to use it in newly diagnosed diabetic children.

To prevent the acute, and almost certainly also the long-term, complications of diabetes, good metabolic control is vital. This depends as much on the diet as on insulin. A carbohydrate-controlled regular diet is therefore essential. The total caloric content should be normal with a high proportion of calories derived from complex carbohydrates, distributed throughout the day in a manner that will "balance" the insulin regimen. The fat content of the diet should be low to reduce atherogenesis.

Metabolic control must be monitored regularly by the parent and/or child by blood and/or urine glucose estimations. Most diabetic children also attend a specialist hospital, but the primary care physician has an important supervisory and supportive role. The education of the patient and the family in the details of day-to-day diabetic management is the cornerstone of successful treatment.

125

Prescribing guidelines and available preparations

Insulin is available in short-, intermediate- and long-acting preparations. Insulin delivery presents problems since it is not possible to mimic either the rapid swings of physiological secretion or delivery directly into the portal circulation.

For acute diabetic ketacidosis, immediate hospital admission is required for rehydration, and soluble insulin (0.1 units/kg per hour) is given by continuous intravenous infusion or frequent intramuscular injections.

For routine replacement, the subcutaneous route is remarkably satisfactory and good glycaemic control can be achieved in most children. New methods of delivery, notably continuous subcutaneous insulin infusion, are being developed.

Establishing therapy

A newly diagnosed and stabilized diabetic child may be started on one or two doses per day of an intermediate-acting human insulin preparation given 15–30 minutes before breakfast and, if necessary, before the evening meal.

As the disease causes progressive destruction of the β cells, it is usually eventually necessary to add a second injection of intermediate-acting insulin before the evening meal, to maintain close control of the blood glucose. A preparation of soluble insulin may be added to the morning dose, and if necessary also to the evening dose, to smooth the insulin delivery and to cover the main meals: this should reduce postprandial hyperglycaemia to a minimum. Mixed preparations are inflexible but ensure consistency.

There is no "correct" dose of insulin. Requirements vary greatly, not only from child to child but also in the same child at different times. Total daily insulin requirements are usually 0.5–1.5 units/kg each day.

Good glycaemic control may be difficult to achieve: many children show sharp swings in blood glucose. These are often best managed by altering the timing and quantity of carbohydrate intake or by exercise rather than by changes in the insulin regimen. Control may be upset by unaccustomed exertion, illness, emotional disturbance and many other factors.

In the treatment of intercurrent illness, preparations with high sugar content should be avoided. Insulin requirements are increased and the insulin dose should never be decreased or stopped. This error has repeatedly proved fatal in childhood diabetes.

Adverse effects

Hypoglycaemia is the major problem. Diabetic children should always carry a readily available source of carbohydrate such as dextrose tablets, boiled sweets or chocolate biscuits. Glucagon is useful in the emergency treatment of hypoglycaemia, given as a single intra-muscular dose of $500\mu g$–1 mg. Parents should learn this technique. Intravenous dextrose 500 mg–1 g/kg over 5 minutes is necessary for severe hypoglycaemia.

Other side effects are now unusual. Although fat atrophy, which was extremely common with previous insulin preparations, does not occur, fat hypertrophy is still sometimes seen. Insulin allergy is now extremely rare.

Drugs for thyroid disorders

Thyroid hormone replacement

Indications for use

Thyroid hormone replacement is used in hypothyroidism. Neonatal screening has shown that congenital hypothyroidism affects about 1 in 4000 infants worldwide, and the incidence of acquired hypothyroidism through childhood is probably similar.

Prescribing guidelines

Although tri-idothyronine is the active hormone physiologically, thyroxine is the preparation of choice for maintenance. Administration of this prohormone permits the peripheral regulatory mechanisms to modulate the production of tri-idothyronine and the alternative inactive thyroxine metabolite, reverse tri-idothyronine, and so provide fine adjustment of the metabolic effect of a given dose.

In acquired hypothyroidism, the correct dose of thyroxine can be judged by reference to the child's own thyroid axis and is defined as the smallest amount that suppresses the plasma thyroid-stimulating hormone (TSH) concentration to the normal range. In congenital hypothyroidism, the feedback loop may be abnormally set and overdosage may result from attempts to suppress fully the TSH.

In both forms of hypothyroidism, a single daily dose of thyroxine of about $100 \mu g / m^2$ (of body surface area) is suitable for all ages. To start with, a daily dose of $8-10 \mu g / kg$ is appropriate in the newborn, $4-5 \mu g / kg$ is usually adequate in children over 1 year and $150-200 \mu g$ when fully grown. Especially in the early months of life when the brain is vulnerable to undertreatment, it is important to check the serum thyroxine regularly, keeping it in the upper part of the normal range for age. Free hormone levels should probably also be in the high normal range. Except in congenital hypothyroidism, it is also useful to check that the TSH is suppressed to the normal range.

Antithyroid drugs

Indications for use

Antithyroid drugs are used for hyperthyroidism (Graves' disease).

Prescribing guidelines and useful drugs

Carbimazole (favoured in Europe) and propylthiouracil (favoured in the United States) are equally effective. Hyperthyroidism is controlled at first by a relatively high dose. When euthyroidism is achieved (usually in 3–6 weeks) a maintenance dose is given, with regular checks on thyroid function. The following doses are suitable for children over 6 years of age.

	Initial dose *(in three divided doses)*	*Maintenance dose* *(in one or two divided doses)*
carbimazole	15 mg/day	5–10 mg/day
propylthiouracil	150 mg/day	50–100 mg/day

In some children, it may be difficult to maintain stable euthyroidism, in which case an alternative approach is to give a higher dose of anti-thyroid drug in combination with a replacement dose of thyroxine. Propranolol may be used to alleviate hyperthyroid symptoms until control is established. The dose is variable owing to a large first-pass effect: 1–4 mg/kg each day in 2–3 divided doses is usually suitable.

The side effects of antithyroid drugs are fairly common, but most are mild. Skin rashes are most frequent; pruritus, urticaria and arthralgia also occur. With mild reactions it is reasonable to try another preparation as cross-sensitivity is rare. Severe reactions are very rare. Agranulocytosis is the most serious; it usually occurs at the start of treatment (but may occur at any time). Monitoring the leucocyte count is often recommended, but is probably of no value. As long as the drug is stopped promptly and the infection is controlled, the prognosis is good. A lupus-like syndrome may also occur and is also an indication to stop medical therapy and use another form of treatment.

Alternatives to drugs

Partial thyroidectomy is required if drug treatment fails or if a relapse occurs when drug treatment is withdrawn after an adequate trial (usually at least 2 years). If surgery is contraindicated, treatment with radio-active iodine can be used.

Note that many surgeons like patients with Graves' disease to be prepared with iodides before surgery to make the gland less vascular. For example, aqueous iodine solution (Lugol's iodine, iodine 5%, potassium iodide 10%) may be given: 1.5 ml/day in three divided doses for 10 days.

Hypothyroidism may result from excess drug use in the treatment of hyperthyroidism (in which case the gland usually enlarges), as part of the natural history of the disease, or following partial thyroidectomy or treatment with iodine-131.

Adrenocorticosteroids

Corticosteroids include those compounds normally secreted by the adrenal cortex as well as synthetic analogues in which some of their physiological actions are enhanced.

Indications for use

Physiological indications are the need to replace absent or inadequate adrenal secretion. This treatment is known as corticosteroid replacement.

Pharmacological indications are the need to control pathological allergic, immune or inflammatory processes. This treatment is known as immunosuppressive and anti-inflammatory therapy.

Although of great therapeutic value, the use of adrenocorticosteroids carries considerable risks, some of which are particularly important in childhood.

Corticosteroid Replacement

The adrenal cortex secretes glucocorticoids (the most important is hydrocortisone), mineralocorticoids (aldosterone is the most active) and weak androgens.

Both primary (Addison's disease) and secondary (adrenocorticotropic hormone (ACTH) deficiency) adrenocortical insufficiency are rare in childhood, but prompt diagnosis and adequate corticosteroid replacement are vital, especially under conditions of stress. If not recognized or treated early enough, they may prove rapidly fatal with hypoglycaemia, salt and water loss, hyperkalaemia and shock.

Replacement is also needed when inadequate secretion results from a block in steroid biosynthesis as in congenital adrenal hyperplasia; in the most common form, 21-hydroxylase deficiency, there is inadequate hydrocortisone production and, in about 50% of these cases, aldosterone deficiency as well.

Prescribing guidelines and useful drugs

For acute adrenal insufficiency

Immediate hospital admission is required, and hydrocortisone sodium succinate 25–100 mg should be given intravenously at once; 25–100 mg should then be given every 4–6 hours (or 50–200 mg/m^2 each day) by continuous intravenous infusion, with adequate fluid replacement as normal saline. At these high doses, the salt-retaining effect of hydrocortisone is adequate, and it is seldom necessary to give parenteral mineralocorticoid, but this can be done with 50–100 mg desoxycortone pivalate given intramuscularly every 2–4 weeks. Desoxycortone acetate (Doca) is no longer widely available.

For chronic adrenal insufficiency

Hydrocortisone (20 mg/m^2 each day or about 600 µg/kg each day) or cortisone (25 mg/m^2 each day or 700 µg/kg each day) is given in at least two doses. Aim to mimic the normal diurnal rhythm by giving the major part (two thirds) in the morning and a smaller dose (one third) in the evening. Adequate replacement (and compliance) can be assessed by checking plasma hydrocortisone levels (and, if available, ACTH levels), ideally obtaining a profile throughout the day.

Mineralocorticoid deficiency is treated with the potent oral salt-retaining compound fludrocortisone (50–200 µg/day in two doses). Added salt is usually not necessary. Hypertension may occur and the blood pressure should be checked regularly.

In congenital adrenal hyperplasia similar steroid doses are needed. Adequate suppression can be checked by measurement of plasma and urinary steroid levels, but growth and bone age are the most important indicators of progress.

Precautionary notes

It is essential that children who require replacement are given parenteral steroids without delay if the oral dose is vomited. The dose must be increased when the child is stressed by illness or trauma, including surgery. Trebling the oral dose is sufficient to cover most illness.

For surgery, hydrocortisone should be given with premedication and by infusion during prolonged operations, and an increased (threefold) maintenance dose should be given parenterally in the immediate postoperative period, returning by decrements to the normal maintenance dose within 2–4 days after uncomplicated operations.

All children on replacement steroids should wear an engraved necklace or bracelet, and every child on steroids for any reason should carry a card giving details of the treatment.

Immunosuppressive and Anti-inflammatory Therapy

There are a number of synthetic fluorinated steroids available that have greatly increased glucocorticoid and anti-inflammatory activity compared with hydrocortisone, but little or no mineralocorticoid activity. The properties of some of these, compared with hydrocortisone, are shown below.

	Potency		
	Glucocorticoid	*Anti-inflammatory*	*Mineralocorticoid*
Glucocorticoids			
hydrocortisone	1	1	1
cortisone	0.8	1	0.8
prednisolone	4	4	0.8
methylprednisolone	5	6	0.5
dexamethasone	30	30	0
Mineralocorticoids			
aldosterone	0.3	9	160
fludrocortisone	80	10	125

Indications for use

Corticosteroids in pharmacological doses may be indicated for the control of a wide variety of allergic and inflammatory diseases, including asthma, nephrotic syndrome, ulcerative colitis and Crohn's disease, juvenile rheumatoid arthritis, collagen disorders, chronic active hepatitis, organ transplant rejection and as adjunctive therapy in the treatment of acute lymphatic leukaemia. Except for asthma, these are all relatively rare disorders for the primary paediatric practitioner and, even in asthma, the use of oral steroids is indicated for fewer than 2% of cases.

In these serious disorders, the correct dose is the least that achieves the desired effect, but the doses that are required are inevitably attended by undesirable side effects and dangers. It is therefore seldom justified to start such treatment without full hospital evaluation and careful consideration of the potential benefits and risks.

Useful drugs

Prednisolone

This is the most widely used corticosteroid in paediatric practice: there are few indications for the use of other compounds. Its glucocorticoid and anti-inflammatory potency is about four times that of hydrocortisone.

The oral dose should initially be 1–2 mg/kg each day, given in two or three doses. It should be reduced as soon as possible to the minimum effective dose. If treatment is continued for more than 4 weeks, use an alternate day regimen if possible. When treatment has continued for more than 2 weeks, the dose should be reduced slowly — 1-mg tablets are useful in this context.

Dexamethasone

This is superior to other steroids in the management of cerebral oedema complicating intracranial lesions, but such treatment should be monitored closely, usually in hospital.

Adrenocorticotropic hormone (ACTH)

ACTH and its synthetic analogue tetracosactide should not be used as alternatives to steroids, as sensitization may occur and their effects are less predictable. They should be reserved for adrenal function testing and for the few conditions in which they may be more effective than prednisolone, such as infantile spasms.

Adverse effects and dangers of steroids

Treatment with supraphysiological doses of steroids for more than a few days inevitably has undesirable effects. In addition, there are a large number of adverse effects that occur less commonly and are related to dosage, duration, age and individual susceptibility. The major problems are the following.

Suppression of endogenous ACTH and adrenal steroid secretion

Increased steroid cover (threefold) is essential during illness and stress. A suppressed state continues for a variable time after cessation of therapy and the child thus remains exposed to the risk of adrenal insufficiency. Steroid cover as above must therefore be given for at least 6 months after any course of steroid therapy sufficient to cause suppression, i.e. when a dose of greater than physiological amounts has been given for more than 2 weeks.

Growth-retarding effect

Glucocorticoids have a potent growth-retarding effect, which is largely caused by the suppression of growth hormone secretion and somatomedin generation. The growth suppression is associated with retardation of skeletal maturation and so, fortunately, there is considerable potential for catch-up growth when treatment has ceased.

Both the adrenal suppression and the effects on growth are minimized by an alternate-day regimen, in which a single dose of prednisolone is given every 48 hours. This permits the recovery of endogenous adrenal axis activity between doses and yet is effective in controlling most disease processes. If it is possible to limit the dose to less than 1 mg/kg every 48 hours, side effects are minimized.

Cushing's syndrome

The main features are weight gain with truncal obesity, "moon face", acne, hirsutism, striae and proximal muscle wasting.

Other adverse effects

Other important but relatively unpredictable side effects include mental effects, commonly euphoria but sometimes depression, diabetes mellitus, peptic ulceration, susceptibility to bacterial infection, impaired wound healing, hypertension, intracranial hypertension, pancreatitis, cataract, Perthes' disease and osteoporosis.

Sex hormones

Hypogonadism

Indications for use

In children with hypogonadism, the replacement of gonadotrophin-releasing hormone, gonadotrophins or gonadal steroids is necessary to induce puberty. In the past, relatively high doses of gonadal steroids were given at relatively late ages, but it is now recognized that it is important to mimic normal physiology more closely; the early changes of puberty occur soon after the age of 11 years in both sexes and take an average 4.5 years to complete. Neither stimulation with hypothalamic-releasing hormones nor full gonadotrophin replacement is yet practicable in routine clinical practice, but the earlier administration of estrogen or testosterone in initially low but increasing doses can induce a more physiological progression of development.

Prescribing guidelines and hormones used

Girls

The preparation of choice is probably ethinylestradiol but natural conjugated estrogens can also be used. Current preparations do not include a unit preparation of ethinylestradiol smaller than $10\mu g$, and fine dose adjustment is therefore difficult. An appropriate initial dose is $2.5-5.0\mu g$/day in one dose. After some months, depending on response, this can be increased to $10\mu g$/day and then to $20-30\mu g$/day in 21-day cycles with a 7-day interval between cycles.

A progesterone such as medroxyprogesterone (5 mg as a single daily dose) should also be given to enhance endometrial shedding, either on the last 7-10 days of the estrogen course or throughout the cycle. For the latter approach, formulations designed for oral contraceptive use — ethinylestradiol ($20\mu g$) with norethisterone acetate (1 mg) or ethinylestradiol ($30\mu g$) with norethisterone ($500\mu g$) — are convenient. Both of these satisfy current recommendations that preparations with low progesterone as well as low estrogen content be given to minimize the risk of carcinogenesis.

135

Boys

The replacement of testosterone is made more difficult because oral preparations of methyltestosterone and its analogues are poorly absorbed and may cause cholestatic jaundice. Intramuscular depot preparations are therefore preferable, e.g. testosterone enantate or mixed testosterone esters (propionate, phenylpropionate, isohexanoate and decanoate). The dose is 50–100 mg given intramuscularly once every 6 weeks, increasing by stages to 250 mg intramuscularly every 3–4 weeks.

Human chorionic gonadotrophin by intramuscular injection once or twice weekly can also be used but, other than causing some testicular enlargement, seems to have no advantages over testosterone.

Cryptorchidism

A course of intramuscular human chorionic gonadotrophin has been reported to induce testicular descent in 15–40% of boys with cryptorchidism, and more recently intranasal gonadotrophin-releasing hormone has been reported to be successful in 10–75%. Some trials, however, have shown that active treatment has little advantage over placebo and it has proved impossible to exclude with certainty all cases of retractile testes. These forms of treatment carry few known risks and may be tried, but if true cryptorchidism, unilateral or bilateral, is confirmed by an experienced person early (preferably before 2 years of age) orchidopexy seems at present the treatment of choice.

Other endocrine agents

Cyproterone

This is an anti-androgen and gonadotrophin-suppressing agent used in the control of precocious puberty in both sexes.

Growth hormone preparations

These preparations, derived from the extraction of human pituitary glands, were highly successful in the treatment of growth failure due to growth hormone deficiency. In 1985, however, after more than 20 years' use of these preparations, four cases of fatal Creutzfeldt-Jakob disease occurred in young people who had previously been treated with human growth hormone. Although cause and effect was not proven, in most countries all human growth hormone preparations have been withdrawn for fear of slow virus contamination. Several biosynthetic preparations are currently on trial and seem effective and safe. They have been licensed in some countries.

Hypothalamic and pituitary hormones

These and their synthetic analogues are widely used in endocrine diagnostic testing and are beginning to find a therapeutic use, such as in the treatment of precocious puberty.

Desmopressin

This is a potent analogue of vasopressin with a prolonged duration of action. It is used for vasopressin replacement in pituitary diabetes insipidus. A solution containing $100\mu g/ml$ is given by intranasal insufflation in a dose of $5-10\mu g$ once or twice daily according to effect.

Malignant disease

Cytotoxic drugs

Cytotoxic drugs should be used only under the supervision of a specialist. Any doctor who is caring for children, however, may from time to time see patients who are receiving these drugs from an oncology clinic. They should not be immunized, particularly with live vaccines. If a child is exposed to measles or chickenpox, advice should be sought from a specialist centre so that appropriate immunoglobulin prophylaxis can be given.

All cytotoxic drugs have important side effects, many of which are unavoidable. It is therefore important to have a knowledge of the major effects of these drugs.

Adverse effects

Bone marrow suppression

Virtually all anticancer agents will suppress the normal bone marrow (the *Vinca* alkaloids are an exception) and cause neutropenia, anaemia and/or thrombocytopenia. Easy bruising and bleeding indicate that the platelet count may be low. The major consequence of a low neutrophil count is that infection, with either common or opportunistic organisms, may rapidly develop and may prove fatal if not treated urgently. Unexplained fever in a potentially neutropenic child is therefore an indication for immediate referral back to the specialist centre. Antibiotics should only be given after consultation with the specialist. Oral *Candida albicans* infection is a common problem, and appropriate antifungal agents can be given (see section on drugs acting on the mouth, p. 167, and section on antifungal drugs, p. 116).

Alopecia

This disappears once therapy has been completed.

Nausea and vomiting

These are common and may be anticipated by children on regular treatment (for prevention, see section on anti-emetics, p. 38).

139

Commonly used drugs and their specific adverse effects

Vinca alkaloids

These include vincristine, vinblastine and vindesine. They can have a neuropathic effect (peripheral and autonomic), usually causing deep tendon reflexes to be lost. Symptomatic manifestations include peripheral paraesthesia, muscle weakness, ptosis, abdominal distension, constipation and jaw pain. Alopecia is another effect.

Alkylating agents

These include cyclophosphamide and ifosfamide. Their adverse effects are haemorrhagic cystitis, sterility (more likely in males and as a late effect) and an increased risk of second tumours.

Anthracyclines

These include doxorubicin. They can have a cardiotoxic effect. This manifests itself as cardiac failure, which occurs in a significant number of patients receiving more than 450 mg/m^2 as a cumulative dose, but is occasionally seen at lower doses.

Bleomycin

Its adverse effects are blistering skin rash and progressive pulmonary fibrosis.

Methotrexate

Its adverse effects are mouth and lower alimentary tract ulceration and neurotoxicity.

Cisplatin

Its adverse effects are severe nausea and vomiting, nephrotoxicity, ototoxicity, peripheral neuropathy, and hypomagnesaemia which may present as tetany.

Terminal care

Terminal illness in children is, surprisingly, often free from pain. The twin objectives of analgesia and mood elevation can be achieved by the use of a narcotic analgesic either on its own or together with a psychotropic drug, such as chlorpromazine.

Methadone has greater mood-elevating properties than other potent analgesics and should be tried first. Give in escalating doses sufficient to keep the child comfortable (see doses for severe pain, p. 99). Morphine is an alternative (see doses for severe pain, p. 99). For bone pain, nonsteroidal anti-inflammatory drugs and steroids may be of value (see p. 155). Pain is most effectively treated by prevention: frequent small doses of analgesics should be given before pain recurs.

It may be necessary to add chlorpromazine to the narcotic analgesic, and an elixir containing 5 mg methadone and 12.5–25 mg chlorpromazine in 5 ml fruit syrup will usually be suitable. The dose or strength can be increased as necessary. It is not necessary to add either cocaine or alcohol to the mixtures.

Parents can be instructed in the technique of intermittent or continuous subcutaneous injection so that they can give strong analgesia with a rapid effect when necessary. The rectal route may be useful for the administration of narcotics.

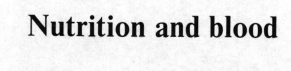

Nutrition and blood

Iron deficiency and treatment

Indications for use

There is no indication for the use of iron or an iron-containing preparation as a nonspecific tonic or appetite stimulant. The only indications for iron use are iron deficiency, usually manifest as hypochromic anaemia, and potential iron deficiency, in which prophylactic iron therapy has been shown to prevent signs of iron deficiency. The indications for iron are:

— dietary iron deficiency;

— prophylaxis in pre-term babies;

— iron deficiency associated with chronic intestinal bleeding due to problems such as salicylate therapy, oesophageal or duodenal ulceration, and hookworm infestation;

— other sources of blood loss, such as menorrhagia; and

— malabsorption syndromes.

Prescribing guidelines

The recommended oral intake of elemental iron is 4.5–6 mg/kg each day and whenever possible this should be accomplished by an adequate dietary intake.

Where dietary supplements are required, there are many preparations available and none has any particular advantage over the others: ferrous sulfate is the cheapest and most commonly used form. Ferrous salts are better absorbed than ferric salts, and there is no indication for the latter. The preparations vary somewhat in the incidence of side effects, although children report fewer problems than adults and side effects are similar for all preparations if related to the elemental iron content of the salt.

There is no need for the concurrent administration of other substances, such as ascorbic acid (to increase iron absorption) or folic acid (as an additional haematinic) unless there are documented mixed deficiencies.

143

When iron is being given for proven iron deficiency, replacement therapy should be continued for at least 3 months after the haemoglobin has returned to normal to ensure that depleted iron stores are replenished.

Start the therapy with ferrous sulfate, and only if adverse effects occur should this be changed. The content of elemental iron should be maintained. The ratio of the amount of elemental iron to ferrous salt is:

Ferrous salt	Elemental Fe (mg)/ferrous salt (mg)
fumarate	0.33
gluconate	0.12
glycine sulfate	0.18
lactate	0.36
succinate	0.35
sulfate	0.20

Adverse effects

Nausea and epigastric pain are related to the elemental iron component and are similar for all preparations. Changes in bowel habit (constipation or diarrhoea) are probably not dose-related but are uncommon in children. Nappies are stained in babies. Stool colour should be very dark, a useful indication of compliance.

Parenteral iron

It is only occasionally necessary to give iron parenterally, e.g. if there is malabsorption or intolerance of iron therapy or if compliance is inadequate. Dosage advice should be sought from a specialist.

Alternatives to drugs

The diet can be improved with iron-containing foods. In certain circumstances, blood transfusions may be necessary. Note that some anaemias do not require iron. For instance, in anaemia associated with infection and inflammation such as arthritis, although the serum iron concentration may be low whole-body iron stores are high, as shown by a normal or elevated serum ferritin level. Other anaemias that do not require iron are thalassaemia, sickle cell anaemia and other haemolytic anaemias (see p. 146), lead poisoning, sideroblastic anaemias and aplastic anaemias (see p. 145).

Other deficiency anaemias

Anaemia may have causes other than iron deficiency, but the institution of alternative haematinic therapy should be undertaken only after full haematological investigation.

Megaloblastic anaemias

These are usually due to a deficiency of folic acid, vitamin B_{12} or both. This may be due to dietary insufficiency or malabsorption resulting from primary bowel disease or, in Scandinavia, from infestation with fish tapeworm. The administration of an anticonvulsant with antifolate action such as phenytoin may also cause this type of anaemia. Note that goats' milk does not contain folic acid or vitamin B_{12}.

	Age	Oral replacement therapy dose	
		Initial	Maintenance
folic acid	< 1 year	500 μg/kg	
	1–4 years	5 mg	1–5 mg per day
	5–12 years	10 mg	

Note that the inappropriate use of folic acid in vitamin B_{12} deficiency may result in progressive and irreversible neurological damage.

The dose of vitamin B_{12} (hydroxocobalamin) for all ages is 30 μg/kg intramuscularly at two- to three-day intervals for five doses, then a maintenance dose of 1 mg every 3 months.

Aplastic anaemia

This condition should be managed by a specialist haematologist.

145

Thalassaemia, sickle cell anaemia and other severe haemolytic anaemias

Because of the rapid turnover of the red cell population in these disorders, folic acid deficiency may become manifest and prophylactic folic acid should be given in all cases.

	Age	Prophylactic dose	
folic acid	< 1 year	250 µg/kg	
	1–4 years	2.5 mg	once daily
	5–12 years	10 mg	

Vitamins

These are widely used as tonics and "pick-me-ups" but there is no evidence that they are of any value.

Indications for use

These include:

— specific deficiency states which are rare in developed countries, apart from B_{12}-deficient megaloblastic anaemia;

— inadequate dietary intake as found, for instance, among Asian groups in the United Kingdom (resulting in rickets), among pre-term babies and among those on special diets (such as for phenylketonuria);

— malabsorption; and

— certain specific metabolic disorders, such as methylmalonic acidaemia.

Classes of vitamin

Vitamin A

Deficiency is rare except in cystic fibrosis. Excessive doses are harmful: they produce dry, rough skin, dry hair, hepatomegaly, and raised intracranial pressure.

Its general use is indicated only in multivitamin preparations for elimination diets, such as in phenylketonuria, or for greater than average requirements, such as in pre-term babies.

Vitamin B complex

Specific B group deficiency is rare in children. B_{12} is required for children with terminal ileum resection or pathology. B_6 (pyridoxine) dependency as a cause of convulsions, and deficiency as a cause of sideroblastic anaemia are rare. No cases of isoniazid-induced peripheral neuropathy have been reported in children, and pyridoxine adjunct therapy during isoniazid treatment of tuberculosis is unnecessary.

Vitamin C

Scurvy due to vitamin C deficiency is extremely rare in children. There is no convincing evidence that vitamin C aids in wound-healing or prevents common colds.

Vitamin D

Vitamin D deficiency is common in Asian children in Europe, and all those under 5 years should be given supplements: ergocalciferol is used.

	Daily dose (all ages)	Indications
ergocalciferol solution (3000 units/ml)	1500–3000 units	rickets
	400–800 units	prevention in high-risk groups (e.g. pre-term babies and Asian children)

Deficiency may be due to malabsorption or chronic liver disease.

In renal osteodystrophy, alfacalcidol or calcitriol should be used as, unlike ergocalciferol, these do not require renal metabolism for conversion to an active form. These preparations are also used in the various forms of vitamin-D-resistant rickets, such as familial hypophosphataemic rickets.

	Indication	Weight of child	Daily dose	
alfacalcidol (drops)	renal osteodystrophy	<20 kg	1 μg/kg	titrate dose to normalize plasma alkaline phosphatase levels
		>20 kg	5 μg/kg	

Calcitriol comes in capsules of 250 ng and 500 ng. The dose is 1–2 μg per day (titrate the dose to normalize plasma alkaline phosphatase levels) for all ages.

Check calcium and phosphate levels regularly; vitamin D preparations combined with calcium should not be used.

Vitamin E

Pre-term babies and patients with cystic fibrosis may require supplementary vitamin E according to specialist advice. Supplements may also be required in steatorrhoea.

Vitamin K

A temporary deficiency of vitamin K sometimes occurs in the newborn, and a single 1-mg dose of phytomenadione is often given.

Children with vitamin K deficiency due to liver disease and mal-absorption may require supplements.

Multivitamin preparations

Pre-term babies require additional vitamins A, C, D and possibly E. Supplements are also required for children on special diets, particularly those that include synthetic amino acid mixtures.

Other drug groups and prescribing situations

Antihistamines

These have limited value in paediatric practice. A large number of H_1-receptor antagonists are available, but they differ little in their pharmacological properties, although they have different durations of action. All have a mild to moderate sedative action, which is a problem in the treatment of allergic symptoms, but can be exploited in specific sedative use, especially in view of the excellent safety record of these drugs.

H_2-receptor antagonists are used primarily in gastro-oesophageal disorders (see p. 48).

Indications for use of H_1-receptor antagonists

For sedation, promethazine and alimemazine (trimeprazine) are the most suitable (see section on sedatives, hypnotics and anxiolytics, p. 81).

For acute and recurrent urticaria, for the relief of symptoms in acute allergic conditions, such as food and drug reactions, and for angio-oedema, chlorphenamine is appropriate (see section on drug therapy for anaphylaxis and angio-oedema, p. 152).

For the prophylaxis and treatment of motion sickness, cinnarizine and cyclizine are satisfactory (see section on anti-emetics, p. 38).

For vomiting due to disease, surgery or drug therapy, pheno-thiazines such as prochlorperazine and perphenazine are most useful (see section on anti-emetics, p. 38).

Note that extrapyramidal effects (dystonic reactions and oculogyric crises) are a particular problem of the phenothiazine group of anti-histamines. They occur less commonly with chlorpromazine, but this is a less effective anti-emetic. These effects may be rapidly stopped by injection of the anticholinergic drug procyclidine or biperiden (see p. 35).

Drug therapy for anaphylaxis and angio-oedema

Acute anaphylaxis

This is rare in childhood, but may result from drugs (especially antibiotics and contrast materials given parenterally), vaccines, hyposensitization preparations, insect stings and food. If it does occur, prompt action may be life-saving:

— the airway should be cleared;

— oxygen should be given if available;

— the child should be laid flat with legs elevated;

— epinephrine (adrenaline) $(1:1000 = 1\,\text{mg/ml})$ should be given immediately by deep intramuscular injection, in a dose of $10\,\mu\text{g}$ $(10\,\mu\text{l})$/kg, to a maximum of $500\,\mu\text{g}$ $(500\,\mu\text{l})$.

If the problem has been caused by injection of an antigen, a similar dose of epinephrine should be given at the site of the injection to retard absorption. An antihistamine (5–10 mg of chlorphenamine) should be given intravenously after the epinephrine. If there is a poor or absent response, the dose of epinephrine can be repeated twice at 15-minute intervals and 5 mg/kg of aminophylline given by slow intravenous injection over 10–20 minutes, continuing with aminophylline by infusion at 1 mg/kg per hour. During this period, immediate referral to hospital is indicated and arrangements for transfer should be made. The physician should accompany the child during transit.

Corticosteroids are too slow-acting to be of value in acute anaphylaxis, but if symptoms persist 50–200 mg of hydrocortisone should be given intravenously.

Precautionary notes

All patients with a previous history of anaphylaxis should wear an engraved bracelet or necklace.

It is wise, especially for those sensitive to insect stings, to carry an emergency kit including a preloaded epinephrine syringe and an antihistamine.

Patients with a previous history of a serious reaction should be considered for desensitization.

Angio-oedema

This results from the exposure of a sensitized patient to an antigen or may be due to a familial condition associated with C1-esterase inhibitor deficiency. As many as 50% of children with acute urticaria may show subcutaneous extension of the oedema (angio-oedema) and in a small number this may involve the larynx or perilaryngeal tissues, so threatening the airway. Intubation or tracheostomy may occasionally be needed. The management of an acute episode otherwise should be as for anaphylaxis.

Drugs used in rheumatic diseases

Arthritis in children is uncommon. The prognosis for both acute and chronic arthritis is generally good, and most children require only simple nonsteroidal anti-inflammatory drugs. Few children need anti-rheumatic agents, most of which have serious adverse effects and should only be used for specific indications. Physical methods of treatment play as important a role as drugs in therapeutic management.

Indications for use

In acute arthritis, it is important to exclude the possibility of acute bacterial infection of bone and/or joints. Most cases will be of the juvenile chronic arthritis type.

Prescribing guidelines

Therapy is symptomatic: to relieve pain and stiffness. Children tend to have less pain than adults, but protective muscle spasm around the joints may occur.

Paracetamol and the narcotic analgesics have no anti-inflammatory activity, and there is no indication to prescribe these.

Most drugs with anti-inflammatory activity differ little in potency. There is marked variation, however, in individual responses to different drugs and also in the incidence of adverse effects. Nearly all drugs may cause gastrointestinal discomfort, usually with nausea and sometimes with bleeding. This can be minimized by taking the drugs after food and trying a variety of formulations to determine which is the most effective and best tolerated by the individual patient. In general, nonsteroidal anti-inflammatory drugs are similar in efficacy to acetylsalicylic acid but have fewer and less severe adverse effects.

Early morning stiffness may be alleviated by using a suppository last thing at night.

Useful drugs

Acetylsalicylic acid

This is cheap but not as well tolerated as other nonsteroidal anti-inflammatory drugs. It has a short half-life and dosing has to be frequent (every 4–6 hours). The oral dose needs to be higher than that for mild pain and antipyresis: 40–90 mg/kg each day in 5–6 divided doses, for all ages. It should be taken after food if possible. Enteric-coated and soluble preparations are preferable.

The measurement of plasma salicylate level is important in providing effective therapy with a minimum of systemic adverse effects (the therapeutic range is 200–300 mg/l). Its adverse effects are gastrointestinal irritation (nausea, vomiting, ulceration, bleeding); tinnitus (difficult to identify in young children); and encephalopathy and hepatotoxicity which occur rarely but should be considered. Regular monitoring is necessary.

Nonsteroidal anti-inflammatory drugs

Although acetylsalicylic acid may be so described, the term "nonsteroidal anti-inflammatory drug" is usually used to describe other drugs. Most are similar in efficacy to acetylsalicylic acid but have fewer and less severe adverse effects. Use with caution in gastric ulceration, oesophageal varices, and renal and hepatic insufficiency. Their adverse effects are gastrointestinal bleeding, ulceration, nausea, vomiting, headache, vertigo and tinnitus. They are generally better tolerated by children than by adults.

In choosing a drug, it may be useful to try several for efficacy and adverse effects. Carefully assess the risk–benefit ratio.

Corticosteroids

These are occasionally indicated, especially in children with severe systemic disturbance. Initially give a short course lasting 3–4 weeks. They may be indicated in iridocyclitis.

Prednisolone should be given: 500 μg–2 mg/kg each day initially in 2–3 divided doses, reducing as soon as possible. Alternate-day therapy should be used if possible (see p. 134).

Adrenocorticotropic hormone is sometimes used: 20 units on alternate days.

For adverse effects and general guidelines, see the section on corticosteroids, p. 130.

Penicillamine, sodium aurothiomalate, chloroquine, hydroxychloroquine

If juvenile chronic arthritis progresses despite appropriate physiotherapy and nonsteroidal anti-inflammatory drug therapy, these drugs may be used. They help about 60% of children over the age of 3 years, but full clinical response may not occur for 4–6 months. The indications

155

and adverse effects are such that specialist advice should always be sought and specific monitoring methods used.

The adverse effects of penicillamine and sodium aurothiomalate are nephritis, marrow suppression, mouth ulcers and rash (which is common). Blood film and urine should be monitored for protein every 4 weeks.

The adverse effects of chloroquine/hydroxychloroquine are retinopathy and rash.

Cytotoxic and immunosuppressive drugs

These should only be used under specialist control. They are rarely indicated except in those children with severe progressive disease which is unresponsive to other measures.

Additional measures

Physiotherapy, hydrotherapy and splinting are as important as drug therapy. A skilled team should provide early and regular supervision.

Therapy for common skin, hair and nail conditions

Both the vehicle and the active ingredient of skin preparations are important, and both often contribute to their effect. The vehicle determines the release and penetration of the active drug, and both the vehicle and the ingredients affect the hydration of the skin. The types of vehicle and main ingredient are discussed first, then a range of preparations are described according to their common indications.

Vehicles

Ointments

These are greasy preparations most suited to chronic dry skin lesion. Most have paraffin bases.

Creams

These are either oily or water-miscible. The latter are easily washed off and acceptable cosmetically.

Lotions

These are suspensions or aqueous solutions that cool inflamed skin by evaporation and allow the active ingredient to spread over large areas.

Pastes

These are stiff preparations with a high percentage of powdered solids. They protect excoriated skin.

Ingredients

Emollients

These hydrate and soothe dry scaly skin, as in ichthyosis and atopic eczema. They include hydrous wool fat, emulsifying wax and paraffins.

157

Barrier creams

These repel moisture and include silicones and castor oil.

Steroid preparations

These suppress inflammatory reactions that are not primarily due to infection. They vary in strength. Use the least potent preparation that is effective so as to minimize adverse effects — this applies especially in infancy when susceptibility to the adverse effects of local steroids is greatest. If applied in large quantities to large areas of skin, especially if the skin is raw and particularly in infants, steroids are systemically absorbed and may cause pituitary–adrenal suppression as well as cushingoid features. Local effects include thinning of the skin and telangiectasia, which may be permanent. The face is particularly vulnerable, and potent steroid applications should be avoided.

Many available preparations include other drugs, especially antibiotic and antifungal agents. The latter are useful, but those containing antibiotics are of limited value and should be avoided because they may encourage colonization with resistant strains of bacteria.

Sensitization to all these products may occur.

Local anaesthetic and antipruritic preparations

Many are available, but all are prone to cause sensitization: they should therefore not be used. Topical steroids have an antipruritic effect, but should not be used for this reason alone.

Cleansing agents

These are important adjuvants in treating skin conditions when soaps prove irritant. Emulsifying ointment is best for scaling disorders, but for weeping areas less irritant preparations such as dilute sodium hypochlorite (in 0.9% saline) are suitable.

Indications for use

Atopic eczema

Controlling the itch and suppressing the desire to scratch are important aspects of therapy. Basic measures are important. Known as "steroid sparing measures" they should reduce and may abolish the need for topical steroid therapy. Use emollient instead of soap for washing; use emollient bath additives when bathing; and use aqueous creams or urea-based emollients (hydrating agents) for dry skin. Use steroids only if these measures fail, and then in the weakest effective preparation. Potent steroids should not be used.

In general, ointments are of greater value than creams in this condition. Occlusive dressings should be avoided. When the condition is chronic and when lichenification is present, ichthammol 1% in an emulsifying ointment, or crude tar 1% or 2% in a zinc ointment or paste may be useful.

It is often necessary to prescribe an oral antihistamine simultaneously. Never use antihistamines topically as they sensitize. Systemic antibiotic therapy is occasionally necessary: secondary infection is usually due to *Staphylococcus aureus* or *Streptococcus pyogenes*.

For management of the infection, use antiseptic baths (either potassium permanganate or chlorhexidine) or an oral antibiotic (flucloxacillin, cloxacillin or erythromycin. A topical antibiotic is best avoided, as it may encourage resistant strains to develop.

Infantile seborrhoeic dermatitis

This is an acute, short-lasting condition in infancy, which is often superinfected with *Candida albicans*. The use of a weak steroid/bacteriostatic/antifungal preparation, such as hydrocortisone 0.5%/chlorhexidine 1%/nystatin 100 000 units/g, hastens recovery. The skin is not itchy so there is no need for systemic antihistamines.

Large, greasy scales on the scalp are easily cleared by 2–5% salicylic acid in aqueous cream applied for 6–8 hours three times a week.

Cradle cap

This can be treated by applying olive oil before using a mild anti-dandruff shampoo, such as one containing cetrimide.

Dandruff

This requires the frequent use of a mild detergent shampoo, such as the widely available commercial preparations containing pyrithione zinc or selenium sulfide.

Nappy rash

Prevention is the best approach. Nappies should be changed frequently and barrier creams, such as dimeticone, and non-occlusive covers should be used where possible. Leaving nappies off in a warm environment helps greatly. Ichthammol preparations, such as ichthammol 1% in zinc ointment, aqueous cream, or zinc oxide cream, are useful for dry lesions. If there is associated candidiasis, see treatment on p. 165.

Psoriasis

Use clean, cosmetically acceptable tar and dithranol preparations, although these are less effective in children than adults. They can be augmented by regular ultraviolet light. Topical steroids should not be used. They may be absorbed and topical side effects are common: striae, skin thinning and telangiectasia. Scalp problems respond to the twice-weekly overnight application of 10–20% salicylic acid in aqueous cream.

Acne

Early onset acne appears to be more severe than that occurring later in adolescence: prompt and effective treatment is necessary to minimize scarring. The skin should be cleansed regularly with a mild detergent solution, such as cetrimide.

Topical therapy. Antiseptic and keratolytic preparations containing benzoyl peroxide or tretinoin are useful. Mild irritation may occur at the start of therapy, but this usually settles rapidly; topical antibiotics are of little value, and topical corticosteroids are contraindicated.

Systemic therapy. Tetracyclines should probably not be used for this condition in those under 8 years of age. Erythromycin is a suitable alternative: long-term low-dose therapy is often effective.

	Initial dose
oxytetracycline	250 mg three times daily before meals for 2–4 weeks
erythromycin	250 mg three times daily for 2–4 weeks

Then reduce to twice daily dosage for maintenance, which can be continued for many months.

Severe acne in girls may respond to the combination of cyproterone 2 mg and ethinylestradiol 50 μg given in 21-day cycles.

Isoretinoin is a new vitamin A derivative for severe cystic acne, but it is teratogenic. Levamisole has also been used. Both these preparations must be used only under close specialist supervision.

160

Plane warts

Most resolve spontaneously in 6–8 months: painful "destructive" therapy is therefore unnecessary. To accelerate resolution, a paint containing salicylic acid or glutaraldehyde may be useful. For resistant problems, carbon dioxide/acetone slush or liquid nitrogen is required: apply every 3 weeks until the warts disappear.

Plantar warts

Some respond to glutaraldehyde or 3–10% formaldehyde in aqueous solution: protect surrounding skin with petroleum jelly and immerse the wart area in the liquid in a shallow trough for 10–15 minutes each night. Isolated stubborn lesions require an application of 25–50% podophyllum in petroleum jelly with occlusion for 1–2 weeks with subsequent curettage of the "debris". This approach is usually painful.

Herpesviral vesicular dermatitis

Most infections require no specific treatment. In primary infections, with herpesviral gingivostomatitis, it is important to maintain adequate hydration, and regular monitoring is needed. In severe cases of herpesviral gingivostomatitis and in eczema herpeticum, use aciclovir.

	Age	Oral dose	
aciclovir	<2 years	100 mg	five times daily at four-hourly intervals for 5 days
	>2 years	200 mg	

Impetigo

The causative organisms are *Staphylococcus aureus* and *Streptococcus pyogenes*. Good hygiene and regular bathing are important, with early attention to minor wounds and abrasions. Local antibiotics are of no value. Treat with oral flucloxacillin or cloxacillin:

Age	Dose	
<1 year	62.5 mg	three times daily for 7 days
1–4 years	125 mg	
5–12 years	250 mg	

More prolonged therapy may be needed in chronic infections. In patients allergic to penicillin, use erythromycin:

Age	Dose	
<1 year	62.5 mg	three times daily for 7 days
1–4 years	125 mg	
5–12 years	250 mg	

161

In recurrent cases, attempt to detect the carrier within the family and treat colonized individuals as for affected children.

Paronychia

Acute infection is usually due to *Staphylococcus aureus*, but may be due to *Streptococcus pyogenes* or human (alpha) herpesvirus 1 or 2. In young children, *Haemophilus influenzae* is occasionally implicated. Chronic infection occurs mainly in adults. In children, infections with *Candida* spp. are an important cause, although gram-negative organisms and *Staphylococcus aureus* are sometimes implicated.

For acute paronychia use oral flucloxacillin or cloxacillin:

Age	Dose	
< 1 year	62.5 mg	
1–4 years	125 mg	three times daily for 7 days
5–12 years	250 mg	

For chronic paronychia take swabs for culture. If candida stomatitis is present, treat with a topical antifungal (see candidiasis, pp. 116 and 165) pending laboratory results.

Erysipelas

This is a rapidly spreading, superficial cellulitis involving the dermis and upper subcutaneous tissues, with involvement of the lymphatics, most commonly caused by *Streptococcus pyogenes*. It should be treated with penicillin G:

Age	Dose	
< 1 year	125 000 units (75 mg)	
1–4 years	250 000 units (150 mg)	six-hourly intravenously or intramuscularly
5–12 years	500 000 units (300 mg)	

When improvement occurs (usually within 24 hours), give phenoxymethylpenicillin:

Age	Oral dose	
< 1 year	62.5 mg	
1–4 years	125 mg	three times daily
5–12 years	250 mg	

162

Review the patient regularly. Admit to hospital if the lesion has extended or the patient's condition has deteriorated.

Other forms of cellulitis

These involve deeper layers of subcutaneous tissues than erysipelas and are characterized by areas of oedema, warmth, tenderness and less marked erythema. There is associated fever and sometimes septicaemia. A wide range of organisms are implicated, especially following trauma. *Staphylococcus aureus* and *Streptococcus pyogenes* are the commonest organisms, but *Haemophilus influenzae* causes cellulitis of the periorbital tissues and cheek, especially in children under 5 years of age.

Note that it may be very difficult to differentiate uncomplicated cellulitis from that associated with underlying bone infection.

Treatment of severe cases.   Where the patient has toxic symptoms or the lesion is rapidly spreading, refer to hospital, but give a single dose of antibiotic if a delay of more than 2 hours is likely.

	Age	Dose	
flucloxacillin	< 1 year	62.5 mg	
	1–4 years	125 mg	intramuscular or intravenous
	5–12 years	250 mg	

For facial cellulitis, give in addition:

	Age	Dose	
ampicillin/amoxicillin	< 1 year	125 mg	
	1–4 years	125 mg	intramuscular or intravenous
	5–12 years	250 mg	

If there is significant local resistance of *Haemophilus influenzae* to ampicillin, use the combination of amoxicillin and clavulanic acid, or cefaclor.

Treatment of mild cases.   Treat with the same antibiotics orally for 7 days. In these cases, review after 24 hours and at intervals thereafter until the cellulitis has completely resolved.

Folliculitis, furunculosis and carbuncles

The causative organism is *Staphylococcus aureus*. Spots and boils originate in the hair follicle, but occasionally the infection spreads to deeper

163

tissues, and to other organs. Soaking the affected area in warm water encourages spontaneous drainage, but large lesions should be incised and drained. If the child has fever or cellulitis, treat with flucloxacillin:

Age	Dose	
<1 year	62.5 mg	
1–4 years	125 mg	three times daily for 7 days
5–12 years	250 mg	

If the patient has toxic symptoms or fever, metastatic spread may have occurred.

When repeated infections occur, neutropenia, a white cell defect or other form of immune deficiency should be considered, but most cases are not associated with a detectable condition. For repeated infections, chlorhexidine or povidone-iodine should be added to the bath water daily to eradicate any *Staphylococcus aureus* carried on the skin and chlorhexidine and neomycin ointment should be applied to the nares three times daily for 14 days.

Traumatic wounds

Wounds and abrasions may become infected with *Staphylococcus aureus* and *Streptococcus* spp. or more rarely with gram-negative organisms. A variety of *Clostridium* spp. that cause gas gangrene, or *C. tetani*, may also be introduced from the environment.

Explore the wound, remove any foreign bodies, excise the devitalized tissue and irrigate the affected area copiously. Early closure should be avoided if there is evidence of environmental contamination.

Patients who have received a primary course of tetanus toxoid should be given a booster dose (but not within 12 months of a previous dose). Other patients should begin a course of three doses immediately.

If there is serious tissue damage or if treatment has been delayed for more than 4 hours, give 250 units of human tetanus antitoxin into the muscle of the opposite limb.

Unless the lesion is a superficial abrasion, give erythromycin, flucloxacillin or cloxacillin orally:

Age	Dose	
<1 year	62.5 mg	
1–4 years	125 mg	three times daily
5–12 years	250 mg	

Human bites

These tend to be infected with more than one type of organism, which may include *Staphylococcus aureus*, aerobic and anaerobic *Streptococcus* spp., spirochaetes and anaerobic gram-negative organisms. Infection may develop rapidly (within 24 hours) with foul-smelling pus. Bites on the hand may give rise to serious problems with rapidly progressive fasciitis.

Proceed as for traumatic wounds above. Primary closure must never be contemplated. Give flucloxacillin or cloxacillin orally as for traumatic wounds.

Animal bites

These are less likely than human bites to become infected, but *Pasteurella multocida* is an important pathogen. Proceed as for traumatic wounds and human bites. Ascertain the occurrence of rabies in the area and, where risk exists, give rabies prophylaxis.

Burns

Minor burns may be treated at home. Infection is usually due to *Staphylococcus aureus*, *Streptococcus pyogenes* or gram-negative organisms. The burn should be covered with a nonadhesive dressing. Sulfadiazine or mafenide cream will reduce the risk of secondary infection. Note that both these agents are contraindicated in sulfonamide hypersensitivity and are occasionally associated with rashes.

Adhesions of the labia minora

This is a common condition of young girls resulting from mild vulvitis and responds well to local therapy. Although generally asymptomatic, it looks strange and is often treated surgically. Application of estrogen cream to the adhesions twice daily for a few days separates them rapidly.

Candidiasis

This is a frequent complication of seborrhoeic eczema and, occasionally, of nappy rash. Nystatin cream and ointment is effective and can be used singly or incorporated in other therapeutic skin preparations. Note that a failure of therapy or a rapid relapse may be due to reinfection from a gastrointestinal reservoir. Oral nystatin may therefore be useful in the treatment of these cases (see p. 116).

Tinea and tinea pedis

Some dermatophytic fungi have an animal source, which should be eradicated. Nylon clothing and tight underwear contribute to sweating and are precipitating factors in tinea affecting the foot and groin. Certain dermatophytes also involve the hair or nails. Oral griseofulvin for 6–8 weeks is recommended for scalp infections, and topical antifungals may reduce spore shedding. Shaving the hair is unnecessary. Nail infections also require oral griseofulvin, but as much as 6–12 months' therapy has sometimes proved unsuccessful. Other infections may be treated with topical agents for 4–6 weeks and certainly for a minimum of 14 days after visible cure (see p. 116).

Dusting powders are ineffective except to combat moisture. Creams should be applied 2–3 times daily. Compound benzoic acid (Whitfield's ointment) is effective, but for cosmetic reasons it is less acceptable in some sites than clotrimazole, econazole or miconazole.

Scabies

The entire family should be treated. Therapeutic agents should be applied to the whole body below the neck. Lotions give easier coverage. Leave for 24 hours and then bathe. Clothes should be changed completely; ordinary laundering is adequate.

Drugs to be used include malathion 0.5%; benzyl benzoate, which is irritant and requires dilution and several applications; and sulfiram which is useful, but parents who consume alcohol may suffer a disulfiram reaction.

Head lice

Because of their longer contact time, lotions are more effective than shampoos. Resistance has rendered lindane less useful than formerly, and resistance also develops to other agents. It is important that application to the area round the ears and neck is not omitted. Carbaril or malathion are the drugs of choice and should be rubbed into dry hair and allowed to dry. The hair should be washed 12 hours later with ordinary shampoo. Dead nits should be removed with a comb. Other members of the family should be checked. Both agents are irritant so avoid the eyes.

Drugs acting on the mouth

Candida stomatitis

This is extremely common in young infants without specific precipitating cause. In children over 1 year, it more usually occurs during acute viral infections or as a sequel to the use of broad spectrum antibiotics. It may also result when feeding teats are improperly sterilized.

Therapeutic failure is more frequent when the period of contact with the antifungal agent is brief: oral infection is best treated with agents left in the mouth after meals or drinks.

For infants, amphotericin B oral paste or miconazole gel is most useful. For older children, amphotericin lozenges or nystatin mixture or pastilles allow long periods of contact between the infection and the therapeutic agent. If all else fails, crystal violet is effective, though messy.

Aphthous ulcers

This is a painful and annoying problem. Treatment, which is not predictably effective, includes carbenoxolone 2% in adhesive base and corticosteroids in lozenges or paste, e.g. triamcinolone acetonide 0.1% (paste) or hydrocortisone sodium succinate (2.5 mg) (lozenges).

Ulcerative gingivitis

This is a common problem often due to anaerobic organisms. It responds poorly to local medication and should be treated with oral phenoxymethylpenicillin or metronidazole, although the latter acts more rapidly.

	Age	Oral dose	
phenoxymethylpenicillin	< 1 year	62.5 mg	
	1–4 years	125 mg	three times daily for 5 days
	5–12 years	250 mg	
metronidazole	< 1 year	50 mg	
	1–4 years	100 mg	three times daily for 3 days
	5–12 years	150–200 mg	

Mouth problems associated with systemic disease or drug use

In Stevens-Johnson syndrome, methotrexate toxicity and other disorders with oral ulceration, local therapy has little specific role, but regular mouth washes are soothing and may help to limit superinfection. Compound thymol glycerin is traditional and pleasant.

In primary severe herpesviral gingivostomatitis, aciclovir may be useful (see p. 161).

Drugs acting on the eye

Infections

To be effective, eye drops must be instilled very frequently, ideally every 10 minutes for the first hour and then hourly (tears dilute or eliminate aqueous solutions).

Ointment is more easily applied than drugs, and contact between the infection and the anti-infective preparation lasts longer.

Preparations containing a corticosteroid as well as an antibacterial agent must be avoided unless the child is under close specialist supervision, as dendritic ulcers, which may be difficult to diagnose, can be made worse.

Bacterial infections

When using antibiotics, it is preferable to prescribe those that are infrequently or never used systemically in order to reduce the possibility of resistance developing. Framycetin (0.5%) or neomycin (0.5%) are traditionally used, and are equally effective and safe. *Staphylococcus aureus* is the commonest infective organism. Severe conjunctivitis may be gonococcal and the patient should be referred immediately. In the newborn and young infants, conjunctivitis that does not respond within 48 hours is likely to be due to *Chlamydia trachomatis* or *Neisseria gonorrhoeae*.

For chlamydial conjunctivitis use tetracycline 1% eye ointment, 4–6 times per day according to effect, together with systemic antibiotic therapy: erythromycin should be given orally, in a dose of 62.5 mg three times daily for 2–3 weeks, for infants under 1 year of age. For suspected gonococcal conjunctivitis, refer immediately to hospital. Investigation of both mother and father is necessary in both of these infections.

Virus infections

Infections with human (alpha) herpesvirus 1 or 2 are best treated with aciclovir 3% ointment every 4 hours.

Ophthalmoscopy

Short-acting, relatively weak mydriatics paralyse the sphincter pupillae sufficiently to facilitate ophthalmoscopy. Homatropine (1% or 2%) and cyclopentolate (0.5% or 1%) drops are preferred for children and act for about 24 hours.

Drugs acting on the external ear

Removal of ear wax

Wax can be softened with sodium bicarbonate ear drops or olive oil. Preparations containing organic solvents are no more effective and may be irritating to the skin of the external auditory meatus. Once wax is softened, it can be removed by syringing.

Otitis externa

This is an eczematous reaction that may become superinfected. Simple cases may respond to syringing or dry mopping. In resistant cases, introduce ribbon gauze soaked in aluminium acetate ear drops 13% or prednisolone drops 0.5%.

When infected, treat with topical antimicrobials (choose an agent that is not used in life-threatening infection, to minimize resistance, such as tetracycline). Apply three times per day for a week. Fungal superinfection is encouraged by prolonged treatment.

Caution must be exercised with polymyxin B and aminoglycosides. They are best avoided if the eardrum is perforated, as they cause deafness in high concentration. Neomycin and framycetin ear drops may lead to sensitization.

INDEX

Entries in **bold type** are names of drugs appearing in the
WHO list of essential drugs

anticonvulsants, 13, 29, 90–97, 145

antidepressant drugs, 11, 84–85

antidiarrhoeal drugs, 42–44

antidotes, 34–35

anti-emetics, 11, 15

antifungal drugs, 75, 116–117, 158–159

antihistamines, 26, 39, 48, 79, 151–153, 159

antihypertensives, 54, 59, 61–62

anti-inflammatory therapy, 132–134

antimalarials, 28, 123–124

antipruritic preparations, 158

antipsychotics, 86–87

antipyretic measures, 56, 92

antipyretics, 11, 55–56, 92

antirheumatic drugs, 154–156

antithyroid drugs, 26, 128–129

antituberculous therapy, 115

antiviral drugs, 118–119

anxiety states, 81

anxiolytics, 83, 151

aphthous ulcers, 167

aplastic anaemia, 145

appetite stimulant drugs, 48

arachis oil, 47

arrhythmias, 49, 85

arthralgia, 129

arthritis, 154–156

arthritis anaemia, 144

Ascaris lumbricoides, 121

ascites, 51

ascorbic acid, 143, 148

asthma, 63–76, 132

ataxia, 94, 96

atopic eczema (dermatitis), 157–159

atropine, 26, 34

attention deficit disorder, 84, 88

azlocillin, 78

bacterial resistance, 169

barbiturates, 34

barrier creams, 158

beclometasone, 62, 75

bed-wetting, 84–85

behavioural effects, 59–60

behaviour modification, 89

benzathine benzylpenicillin, 16, 109

benzodiazepines, 82–83, 91–93, 96–97

benzoic acid, 166

benzoyl peroxide, 160

benzyl benzoate, 166

bephenium, 121

β_2-adrenergic agonist drugs, 15, 63–68, 74–77

β-adrenergic blocking drugs, 26, 102

β-lactamase enzymes, 110

betamethasone, 62, 75

biliary colic, 99

bioavailability, 7, 15

biotransformation, 8, 9

biperiden, 35, 151

bisacodyl, 47

bites, 165

bleomycin, 140

blood, 143

blood–brain barrier, 8

body fluids, 8

bone and joint infection, 105–106, 154

bone marrow suppression, 105, 139–140, 156

bone pain, 141

Bordetella pertussis, 105, 112

boric acid, 15

bradyarrhythmias, 50

bradycardia, 26

bran, 46

breastfeeding, 25–26

breast-milk, 25–26

bromocriptine, 26

bronchiectasis, 113

bronchodilator drugs, 63–67

Brucella spp., 104

combination products, 13, 100
combination therapy, 22
common cold, 148
compliance, 5, 13–14, 18, 22, 92
compound thymol glycerin, 168
concentration, 16, 18, 21–22, 27, 50, 69, 92–96
  breast-milk, 25–26
  carbamazepine, 94
  digoxin, 50
  ethosuximide, 96
  fluctuation in, 18, 21–22, 69, 94
  phenobarbital, 95
  phenytoin, 96
  steady state, 18, 21
  theophylline, 69
conduct disorders, 86
congenital hypothyroidism, 128
conjugation, 8
conjunctivitis, 169
constipation, 45, 62, 74, 85, 99, 140, 144
convulsions, 90–97
corticosteroids, 15, 26–27, 74–76, 130–134, 141, 152–153, 155, 158–160, 167, 169
cortisone, 131–134
co-trimoxazole, 106, 111–112
cough suppressants, 13, 57, 112
cradle cap, 159
creams, 157–160, 166
Creutzfeldt-Jakob disease, 137
Crohn's disease, 43, 132
cromoglicate disodium, 15, 61, 63, 66, 74, 77
croup, 112
crude tar, 159
crystal violet, 166
cushingoid features, 75, 158
Cushing's syndrome, 134
cutaneous larva migrans, 122
cyanosis, 77
cyclizine, 39, 151
cyclopentolate, 170

cyclophosphamide, 140
cyproterone, 137, 160
cystic fibrosis, 78–79, 105, 113, 147
cytochrome P450, 8
cytotoxic drugs, 27, 38, 83, 139–140, 156

dandruff, 159
dapsone, 28, 123–124
deafness as adverse effect of furosemide/aminoglycosides, 52
decongestants, 11, 13, 59–60, 111
dendritic ulcers, 169
dependence, 99
depression, 84, 134
dermatophytic fungi, 116–117, 166
desensitization, 76, 153
desensitizing injections, 61–62, 76
desmopressin, 137
desoxycortone acetate, 131
desoxycortone pivalate, 131
dexamethasone, 132–133
dexamphetamine, 89
diabetes insipidus, 137
diabetes mellitus, 84, 125–127, 134
diarrhoea, 42–43, 144
diazepam, 15, 83, 91–92, 97
diazoxide, 26
dicloxacillin, 104
dicycloverine, 41
diethylstilbestrol, 28
digoxin, 10, 15, 23, 35, 50
  binding sites, 10
  concentration monitoring, 50
  poisoning, 35
  toxicity, 50
dihydrocodeine tartrate, 98
dimenhydrinate, 39
diphenoxylate, 35, 43
diphenylbutylpiperidines, 87
diprophylline, 69
disaccharide intolerance, 43

178

179

ipecacuanha, 34, 58
ipratropium bromide, 74
iron, 143–144
irritability, 10
irritable bowel syndrome, 41
irritant injections, 74
irritants, 15
isoniazid, 26, 29, 107, 114, 147
isoprenaline, 65
isoretinoin, 160
ispaghul husk, 46

jaw pain, 140
juvenile chronic arthritis, 132, 154–156

kaolin mixture, paediatric, 43
keratolytic preparations, 160
ketoconazole, 117
ketogenic diet, 93
Klebsiella spp., 104

labelling, 14
labia minora adhesions, 165
lactose in medicines, 14
lactulose, 46
larva migrans, 122
latamoxef, 29, 95
laxatives, 42, 45–47
Legionella pneumophila, 105
levamizole, 160
lice, head, 166
lincomycin, 105
linctus codeine, 57
linctus, noscapine, 57
lindane, 166
liquid nitrogen, 161
liquid paraffin, 47
liquid preparations, 14
lithium, 26
liver, 8
local anaesthetics, 158
loperamide, 43–44

lorazepam, 83
lotions, 157
lupus-like syndrome, 129

mafenide, 28, 165
magnesium trisilicate, 37
malabsorption, 79, 145, 147
malabsorption syndrome, 43, 143
malathion, 166
malignant disease, 139
mania, 85
mannitol, 53
marrow suppression, bone, 105, 139–140, 156
mast cell stabilizers, 61
measles, 139
mebendazole, 120–121
medicalization, 5, 11
medroxyprogesterone, 135
megacolon, 45
megaloblastic anaemia, 145, 147
membrane penetration, 8
meningococcal infections, 106
menorrhagia, 143
metabolic rate, 8
metabolism, first-pass, 7, 74
metabolites, active, 22
methadone, 99, 141
methotrexate, 140
methotrexate toxicity, 168
methylmalonic acidaemia, 147
methylphenidate, 88–89
methylprednisolone, 132
methyltestosterone, 136
methysergide, 102
metoclopramide, 27, 34–35, 41, 100–101
metronidazole, 15, 29, 95, 106, 120, 167
miconazole, 117, 166–167
microsomal enzyme system, 8
microspherules, 79
Microsporum spp., 116

180

migraine, 38, 100–102
migraine trigger factors, 101
mineralocorticoid deficiency, 131
"moon face", 134
morphine, 35, 99, 141
motion sickness, 38, 151
mouth, drugs acting on, 167
mouth ulcers, 140
mucolytics, 58, 78
mucosal oedema, nasal, 59
multivitamin preparations, 149
muscle spasm, 154
muscle weakness, 140
Mycobacterium tuberculosis, 105
Mycoplasma pneumoniae, 105, 113

nalidixic acid, 26
nappy rash, 15, 159, 165
narcotics, 26, 141, 154
nasal obstruction, 59
nausea, 116, 120, 124, 139–140, 144, 154–156
nebulized drugs, 66–68, 74–75, 78
Necator spp., 121
Neisseria gonorrhoeae, 169
Neisseria meningitidis, 106
Neisseria spp., 104
neomycin, 105–106, 164, 169, 171
nephritis, 156
nephrotic syndrome, 51–52, 132
nephrotoxicity, 105, 140
neurotoxicity, 140
neutropenia, 139, 164
niclosamide, 122
nitrazepam, 82
nitrofurans, 28
nitrofurantoin, 28, 106
nonsteroidal anti-inflammatory agents, 26, 141, 154
norethisterone acetate, 135

Norisen Grass, 62
noscapine linctus, 57
nutrition, 143
nystagmus, 96
nystatin, 116–117, 159, 165, 167

obesity, 86
occlusive dressings, 159
oculogyric crises, 35, 151
oedema, 51
oesophagitis, 37
ointments, 157
olive oil, 159, 171
opiate analogues, 112
opiates, 38
optic neuritis, 107
oral replacement fluids, 43
oral route, 13
oral steroids, 67
oral ulceration, 167–168
oranges, in migraine, 101
orciprenaline, 65
organic solvents, 171
osmotic diuretics, 46, 53
osteoporosis, 134
otitis externa, 171
otitis media, 55, 111
ototoxicity 105, 140
overprescribing, 6
oxidation, 8
oxymetazoline, 59
oxytetracycline, 160

paediatric kaolin mixture, 43
pancreatic enzymes, 78–79
pancreatitis, 134
paracetamol, 15, 56, 98, 100, 102, 154
paraffins, 157
paraldehyde, 15, 91
parasympathomimetic agents, 10
paronychia, 162

pastes, 157
Pasteurella multocida, 165
penicillamine, 155
penicillin G, 104, 162
penicillins, 9, 16, 104, 109
peptic ulcer, 37, 41, 48, 134
perfusion, organ, 78
periciazine, 86
peripheral neuropathy, 107, 140, 147
peripheral paraesthesia, 140
perphenazine, 39, 86, 151
Perthes' disease, 134
pertussis, 112
pethidine, 99
petroleum jelly, 161
petroleum products, 35
pharmacodynamics, 7, 9
pharmacokinetics, 7, 12
pheneticillin,16, 104, 113
phenindione, 26
phenobarbital, 10, 22–23, 29, 91–93, 95, 112
phenobarbital–chloramphenicol interaction, 29
phenothiazines, 10, 16, 27, 34–35, 83, 86–87, 99, 151
phenoxymethylpenicillin, 16, 104, 108–110, 113, 162, 167
phenylethylmalonamide, 22
phenylketonuria, 147
phenytoin, 15, 23, 29, 91–92, 95–96, 145
phosphate enemas, 47
photosensitivity, 116
physiotherapy, 78, 156
phytomenadione, 148
pimozide, 87
piperacillin, 78
piperazine, 120–121
pirbuterol, 70
pizotifen, 102
plane warts, 161
plantar warts, 161
Plasmodium falciparum, 123

Plasmodium vivax, 123–124
pneumococcal vaccine, 110
pneumonia, 113
podophyllum, 161
poisoning, 34–35
pollinosis, 61
polymyxin B, 171
potassium, 51
potassium-losing diuretics, 51–52
potassium permanganate, 159
potassium-sparing diuretics, 13, 51, 53
potassium supplements, 51–53
povidone-iodine, 164
precocious puberty, 137
prednisolone, 68, 75–76, 132–134, 155, 171
premedication, 81
prescriber, 5, 14, 21, 31
prescribing, 10, 14, 31
pre-term babies, 147–149
primaquine, 28
primidone, 22, 96
prochlorperazine, 39, 86, 151
procyclidine, 35, 151
proguanil, 123–124
promazine, 86
promethazine, 83, 151
prophylactic drugs, 74
prophylaxis, 15–16, 107
  bowel, 106
  endocarditis, 109
  Haemophilus influenzae, 108
  herpetic infections, 118
  iron therapy, 143
  malaria, 123–124
  meningococcal infection, 107–108
  rheumatic fever, 108–109
  sickle cell disease, 110
  splenectomy, 110
  Streptococcus pneumoniae, 110
  urinary tract infection, 114
propranolol, 102, 129

182

tinnitus, 155
tixocortol, 62
tobramycin, 78
tolerance, 84, 88, 97, 99
tooth staining, 27, 104
topical antibiotics, 159, 171
topical steroids, inhalation, 61–62, 67, 74–76
toxicity, 12, 15
Toxocara spp., 122
tracheostomy, 153
traumatic wounds, 164
tretinoin, 160
triamcinolone acetonide, 167
triamterine, 53
trichinosis, 122
Trichophyton spp., 116
Trichuris trichuria, 121
tricyclic antidepressants, 11, 35, 84–85, 88–89
tri-iodothyronine, 128
trimeprazine, 10, 82–83, 151
trimethoprim, 106, 113–114
tuberculosis, 106, 114–115, 147
tubular secretion, 9

ulcerative colitis, 132
ulcer-healing drugs, 48
urinary tract infection, 85, 104, 106, 113–114
urine, darkening of, 120
urticaria, 107, 151, 153

vasopressin, 137
vehicles for skin medication, 157
ventricular tachycardia, 49, 54
vertigo, 155
vidarabine, 118–119
vinblastine, 140
vinca alkaloids, 140
vincristine, 140
vindesine, 140

visceral larva migrans, 122
vitamin A derivatives, 160
vitamin B_6, 147
vitamin B_{12}, 145
vitamin C, 28, 143, 148
vitamin D, 148
vitamin E, 148
vitamin K, 148–149
vitamins, 28, 79
vitamin supplements, 78–79, 147–149
volume of distribution, 8
vomiting, 99, 139–140
vulvitis, 165

warfarin, 26
warts, 161
water-soluble drugs, 8
Whitfield's ointment, 166
"worm wobble", 121

xanthine derivatives, 69
xylometazoline hydrochloride, 59

zinc oxide cream, 160
zoster, 118
zoster ocular disease, 118

WHO publications may be obtained, direct or through booksellers, from:

ALGERIA: Entreprise nationale du Livre (ENAL), 3 bd Zirout Youcef, ALGIERS

ARGENTINA: Carlos Hirsch, SRL, Florida 165, Galerías Güemes, Escritorio 453/465, BUENOS AIRES

AUSTRALIA: Hunter Publications, 58A Gipps Street, COLLINGWOOD, VIC 3066 — Australian Government Publishing Service *(Mail order sales)*, P.O. Box 84, CANBERRA A.C.T. 2601; *or over the counter from:* Australian Government Publishing Service Bookshops *at:* 70 Alinga Street, CANBERRA CITY A.C.T. 2600; 294 Adelaide Street, BRISBANE, Queensland 4000; 347 Swanston Street, MELBOURNE, VIC 3000; 309 Pitt Street, SYDNEY, N.S.W. 2000; Mt Newman House, 200 St. George's Terrace, PERTH, WA 6000; Industry House, 12 Pirie Street, ADELAID, SA 5000; 156–162 Macquarie Street, HOBART, TAS 7000 — R. Hill & Son Ltd., 608 St. Kilda Road, MELBOURNE, VIC 3004; Lawson House, 10–12 Clark Street, CROW'S NEST, NSW 2065

AUSTRIA: Gerold & Co., Graben 31, 1011 VIENNA I

BANGLADESH: The WHO Representative, G.P.O. Box 250, DHAKA 5

BELGIUM: *For books:* Office International de Librairie s.a., avenue Marnix 30, 1050 BRUSSELS. *For periodicals and subscriptions:* Office International des Périodiques, avenue Louise 485, 1050 BRUSSELS — *Subscriptions to World Health only:* Jean de Lannoy, 202 avenue du Roi, 1060 BRUSSELS

BHUTAN: *see* India, WHO Regional Office

BOTSWANA: Botsalo Books (Pty) Ltd., P.O. Box 1532, GABORONE

BRAZIL: Centro Latinoamericano de Informação em Ciencias de Saúde (BIREME), Organização Panamericana de Saúde, Sector de Publicações, C.P. 20381 - Rua Botucatu 862, 04023 SÃO PAULO, SP

BURMA: *see* India, WHO Regional Office

CANADA: Canadian Public Health Association, 1335 Carling Avenue, Suite 210, OTTAWA, Ont. K1Z 8N8. (Tel: (613) 725–3769. Telex: 21–053–3841)

CHINA: China National Publications Import & Export Corporation, P.O. Box 88, BEIJING (PEKING)

DEMOCRATIC PEOPLE'S REPUBLIC OF KOREA: *see* India, WHO Regional Office

DENMARK: Munksgaard Export and Subscription Service, Nørre Søgade 35, 1370 COPENHAGEN K (Tel: + 45 1 12 85 70)

FIJI: The WHO Representative, P.O. Box 113, SUVA

FINLAND: Akateeminen Kirjakauppa, Keskuskatu 2, 00101 HELSINKI 10

FRANCE: Librairie Arnette, 2 rue Casimir-Delavigne, 75006 PARIS

GERMAN DEMOCRATIC REPUBLIC: Buchhaus Leipzig, Postfach 140, 701 LEIPZIG

GERMANY FEDERAL REPUBLIC OF: Govi-Verlag GmbH, Ginnheimerstrasse 20, Postfach 5360, 6236 ESCHBORN — Buchhandlung Alexander Horn, Friedrichstrasse 39, Postfach 3340, 6200 WIESBADEN

GHANA: Fides Enterprises, P.O. Box 1628, ACCRA

GREECE: G.C. Eleftheroudakis S.A., Librairie internationale, rue Nikis 4, ATHENS (T. 126)

HONG KONG: Hong Kong Government Information Services, Beaconsfield House, 6th Floor, Queen's Road, Central, VICTORIA

HUNGARY: Kultura, P.O.B. 149, BUDAPEST 62

INDIA: WHO Regional Office for South-East Asia, World Health House, Indraprastha Estate, Mahatma Gandhi Road, NEW DELHI 110002

INDONESIA: P.T. Kalman Media Pusaka, Pusat Perdagangan Senen, Block I, 4th Floor, P.O. Box 3433/Jkt, JAKARTA

IRAN (ISLAMIC REPUBLIC OF): Iran University Press, 85 Park Avenue, P.O. Box 54/551, TEHERAN

IRELAND: TDC Publishers, 12 North Frederick Street, DUBLIN 1 (Tel: 744835–749677)

ISRAEL: Heiliger & Co., 3 Nathan Strauss Street, JERUSALEM 94227

ITALY: Edizioni Minerva Medica, Corso Bramante 83–85, 10126 TURIN; Via Lamarmora 3, 20100 MILAN; Via Spallanzani 9, 00161 ROME

JAPAN: Maruzen Co. Ltd., P.O. Box 5050, TOKYO International, 100–31

JORDAN: Jordan Book Centre Co. Ltd., University Street, P.O. Box 301 (Al-Jubeiha), AMMAN

KUWAIT: The Kuwait Bookshops Co. Ltd., Thunayan Al-Ghanem Bldg, P.O. Box 2942, KUWAIT

LAO PEOPLE'S DEMOCRATIC REPUBLIC: The WHO Representative, P.O. Box 343, VIENTIANE

LUXEMBOURG: Librairie du Centre, 49 bd Royal, LUXEMBOURG

MALAWI: Malawi Book Service, P.O. Box 30044, Chichiti, BLANTYRE 3